Nutrition for Dance and Performance

Nutrition for Dance and Performance is the first complete textbook written by an experienced dietitian specialising in the field of dance nutrition. It seeks to provide both dancers-in-training and instructors with practical advice on dance nutrition for health and performance. It is also highly relevant for dance professionals. With an in-depth and extensive coverage on all nutrition topics relevant to dancers, this book covers nutrition for the scenarios dancers face, including day-to-day training and rehearsals, peak performance, injuries, immunonutrition, nutrition and stress management. Information is included on topics applicable to individual dancers including advice for dancers with Type 1 diabetes and clinical conditions relating to gut health.

The book guides the reader through the macronutrients making up the diet, their chemical structure and their role in health and optimal performance. Readers are shown how to estimate energy and nutrient needs based on their schedule, type of dance undertaken and personal goals before considering the practical aspects of dance nutrition; from nutrition planning to dietary supplements, strategies for assessing the need to alter body composition and guidance on undertaking health-focused changes.

Nutrition for Dance and Performance combines and condenses the author's knowledge and many years of experience working in the dance industry to translate nutrition science into a practical guide. Bringing together the latest research in dance science and nutrition, this book aims to be a trusted reference and practical textbook for students of Dance, Dance Nutrition, Dance Performance, Sport Nutrition and Sport Science more generally as well as for those training in the dance industry, dance teachers and professionals.

Jasmine Challis is a freelance Registered Nutritionist (UK Association for Nutrition) and Dietitian registered with the Health Care Professions Council, and is on the UK Sport and Exercise Nutrition Register (SENR) focussing on dance. She completed an MRes in Sport and Exercise Science in 2018. She is on the Dance Medicine and Science Expert Panel for One Dance UK and is on the board of The Bridge Dance Project. She has worked across the dance field for over 30 years giving talks, running workshops and providing 1:1 sessions for dancers and dance students.

Nutrition for Dance and Performance

Jasmine Challis

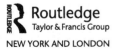 Routledge
Taylor & Francis Group

NEW YORK AND LONDON

Designed cover image: dancer image: StudioM1
Food image: fcafotodigital

First published 2023
by Routledge
605 Third Avenue, New York, NY 10158

and by Routledge
4 Park Square, Milton Park, Abingdon, Oxon, OX14 4RN

Routledge is an imprint of the Taylor & Francis Group, an informa business

ISBN: 978-1-032-11243-5 (hbk)
ISBN: 978-1-032-11242-8 (pbk)
ISBN: 978-1-003-21900-2 (ebk)

DOI: 10.4324/9781003219002

Typeset in Times New Roman
by codeMantra

Contents

Contents

12 Plant-based diets for dancers 222

13 Clinical nutrition 242

Appendix A: Glossary of micronutrients: minerals and
                          vitamins 261
Appendix B: Recipes 271
Glossary 299
Index 301

Foreword

Dancers are athletes and should be treated as such. Yet in-depth understanding of the role of nutrition as a real and important performance aid for dancers is lacking. Good nutrition is essential to the optimisation of a dancer's training, rehearsal and performance. *Nutrition for Dance and Performance* is a must-read for student and professional dancers as well as school and company teachers and managers.

Each chapter provides useful myth-busters, further resources and learning outcomes, underpinned by sound theory. Packed full of practical suggestions, this is a *when, why and what to eat* book for dancers of any style or genre.

Jasmine Challis gives us an excellent, easy-to-read, evidence-based resource, which contains not only fundamental information about metabolism, macronutrients, supplements, hydration and allergies, but helpful tips on what and when to eat, during a dancer's busy schedule and in accordance with the varying demands of dance activity.

This is the first comprehensive book of its kind, written by one of the most acclaimed nutritionist-researchers in dance. It is a resource the dance world has been calling for – the wait is finally over.

Professor Emma Redding MBE, PhD
Director | Victorian College of the Arts
Past-President International Association for Dance Medicine and Science

Preface

Welcome to *Nutrition for Dance and Performance*, a new book, which covers both the theory of major topics of nutrition relevant to dancers, and how this translates practically into food and drink.

Although the chapters do flow from one topic to the next, they are designed to stand alone as far as is possible. Direction is given to other chapters where topics straddle across two chapters, which is somewhat inevitable with nutrition. Feel free to start wherever seems most useful. I very much hope the information will support you to identify and meet your nutritional goals for training, rehearsals and performance.

There is of course, more that I would have liked to have included, but was not able to fit in. The references and resources will guide you to more information on most topics, as will your own individual research.

A quick final note before leaving you to explore the fabulous world of nutrition: I am very aware that some dancers prefer not to be faced with numbers, in particular calories, a measure of the energy content in food and energy used in life. While energy is discussed, and numerical information included, nutrition is so much more than calories, and guidance is given to those who prefer to avoid numerical detail.

Jasmine Challis

Author

Jasmine Challis BSc MRes RD (SENR)
Jasmine is an Accredited Nutritionist and Dietitian on the UK Sport and Exercise Nutrition Register (SENR) focussing on dance. She has worked across the dance field for over 30 years giving talks and running workshops for dance students, dancers and dance teachers, and providing 1:1 sessions for dancers and dance students. She is nutrition consultant for the Dance UK Information Nutrition for Dancers and is co-author of the International Association for Dance Medicine and Science (IADMS) Nutrition Resource Paper (2016), as well as the Nutrition chapters in a number of dancer health books. She is on the board of The Bridge Dance Project. She has presented at the IADMS annual conference regularly. She completed an MRes in Sport and Exercise Science (with distinction) in 2018, her research project was with Irish dancers. She also works with circus performers and acting/technical students, has contributed to medical and dietetic textbooks and continues working clinically mainly with those suffering from eating disorders.

Acknowledgements

This book would not have been written without the help of many people. If I have forgotten anyone, my apologies, please know your time and efforts were very much appreciated. It has certainly felt like a team effort to get to the final manuscript, and everyone who has contributed has given their time, skills and energy very generously.

I am extremely grateful to Kathryn Peters, who gave invaluable feedback on two chapters, sourced some of the fabulous dancer photographs, devised some of the figures, and, together with Francesca Straniero, assembled the recipes section in a very short time frame.

My very deep appreciation to the colleagues and friends who gave invaluable feedback on individual chapters: Talia Cecchele, Stephanie De'Ath, Claire Farmer, Kim Hutt, Dr Siobhan Mitchell, Dr Stephanie Potrek (AusDancers Overseas), Monika Saigal and Dr Margaret Wilson. I thank you all for your generous support.

Special thanks to Zerlina Mastin, who had a major role in drafting the original proposal, and also gave initial feedback, reviewed two chapters, gave suggestions for photographs and provided support throughout the creation process.

I am very grateful to my family who have contributed feedback and suggestions along the way: Dave, Tom, Jodie, Sam and Lucy, many thanks to you all for your input and support.

Photographers: Jon Applegate, Robert Biesemans, Dani Bower, Mike Cooper, Arthur Giglioli, Anna Moutou, Helen Rimmell and Steve Scaddon: thank you all for allowing me to use your wonderful photos.

Recipe photos are courtesy of Francesca Straniero, Kathryn Peters, plus myself.

The dancers: Nefeli 'sMash' Tsiouti PT, MA, MSc, Founder of Project Breakalign; Isabella Gasparini & Paulo Rodrigues; Helen, Xena, Serena, Sam, Zeb, Rebecca, Tom, Billy, Steven, Dean, Alexander, Jess, Richard, Aila and Cristi: thank you all for bringing your skills, energy and passion for dance to the book.

Thanks to Erin Sanchez and Dani Bower at One Dance UK for help with sourcing dancer photos.

Thanks also to Professor Emma Redding for finding time to write a wonderful foreword.

Last, but not least, thanks to the reviewers of the original proposal who supported it, and to the team at Taylor & Francis Group for their support through the process.

Please note: where photographs are not credited to the photographers above, or as stock images, they are my own.

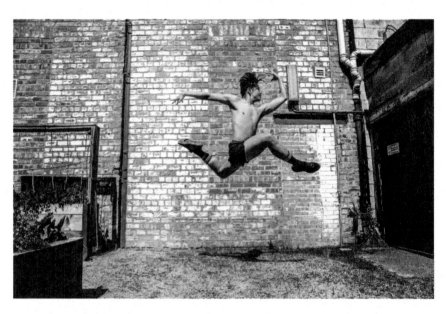

Photo 1.1 To soar through the air the dancer relies on nutrients consumed previously.
Source: Photo courtesy of Dani Bower photography.

1 Dance nutrition

Contents

I Introduction

The art of dance is physically demanding on the whole body but particularly on the musculoskeletal system. For the dancer as a performing artist, artistry and expression are primary goals, but unless dancers are physiologically honed to the same extent as they are artistically, their physical conditioning may potentially be the limiting factor in their development and performance. Physiological training of today's dancers is evolving as the art form itself evolves. The performing artist's body is their unique instrument which is the foundation for performance. And that instrument requires energy and nutrients to perform.

Historically nutrition was regarded as both an art and a science, as evidenced by a textbook from 1944 entitled 'The Art and Science of Nutrition: a Textbook on the Theory and Application of Nutrition' by Hawley and Carden. Today, nutrition is more regarded as a science, but there is a definite art to interpreting and translating the science into practical recommendations that are meaningful for individuals, which is the role of the dietitian. In fact, nutrition is underpinned by the sciences of biology, chemistry, biochemistry, microbiology, physiology and psychology, the last of which is itself is often regarded as being a combination of science and art. As a relatively young

DOI: 10.4324/9781003219002-1

science, nutrition is still evolving as research provides insights into how the human body best functions, which can be of use to the dancer.

There are many factors that propel a dancer to a successful career: focus, musicality and spatial awareness, genetics, training, determination and hard work. Nutrition is also a crucial contributor to optimal dance performance. Sometimes nutrition is overlooked because genetics and/or training plus determination have carried the dancer through despite a lacklustre nutritional plan. Only at the highest levels of performance and competition will weakness(es) in any of these departments be exposed. Therefore, to achieve optimal results, nutrition should be emphasised in the same way that talent and a properly designed training/practice plan are viewed.

II Nutrition and the dancer

Appropriate nutrition forms the foundation upon which dance performance is built. A good nutrition program supports every aspect of physical and mental abilities. Everything from your level of hydration to the timing of your carbohydrate intake will impact on your performance. Your muscles need to be maintained and potentially become stronger with adequate protein and appropriate strength training. Your ability to sustain the intermittently high-intensity workload that characterises dance is highly dependent on your glycogen stores. Nutrition fuels dance performance – there is no other source of energy for humans. Good nutrition can also be a major contributor to reducing fatigue, injury risk and poor recovery, all three of which can hinder how well a dancer performs, and how quickly they can return to the stage. There is also a psychological component – nutrition contributes to mental as well as physical well-being in combination with other strategies such as training optimisation, programmed rest, recovery techniques and stress management. A healthy diet and a performance diet are synonymous with one another.

But dance nutrition is of course far more than hydration, carbohydrates to fuel activity and protein for mending muscles. All of the vitamins and minerals identified as requirements for the human body play a role in helping your body to be the best it can be. Calcium and vitamin D for bone health, adequate iron, vitamin B12 and folate to prevent fatigue and antioxidants to support the immune system are only a few roles nutrition plays in sustaining the healthy dancer.

Figure 1.1 shows the organ systems of the body. Nutrition is crucial for every system to function optimally. For example, vitamins such as folate and B12 (types of 'B complex' vitamin) support the healthy function of the nervous system (the brain, the spinal cord and the nerves). A deficiency in either of these vitamins can cause a wide range of problems, including vision problems, memory problems, fatigue and loss of physical coordination. Every body system can and will be affected by nutrient deficiencies.

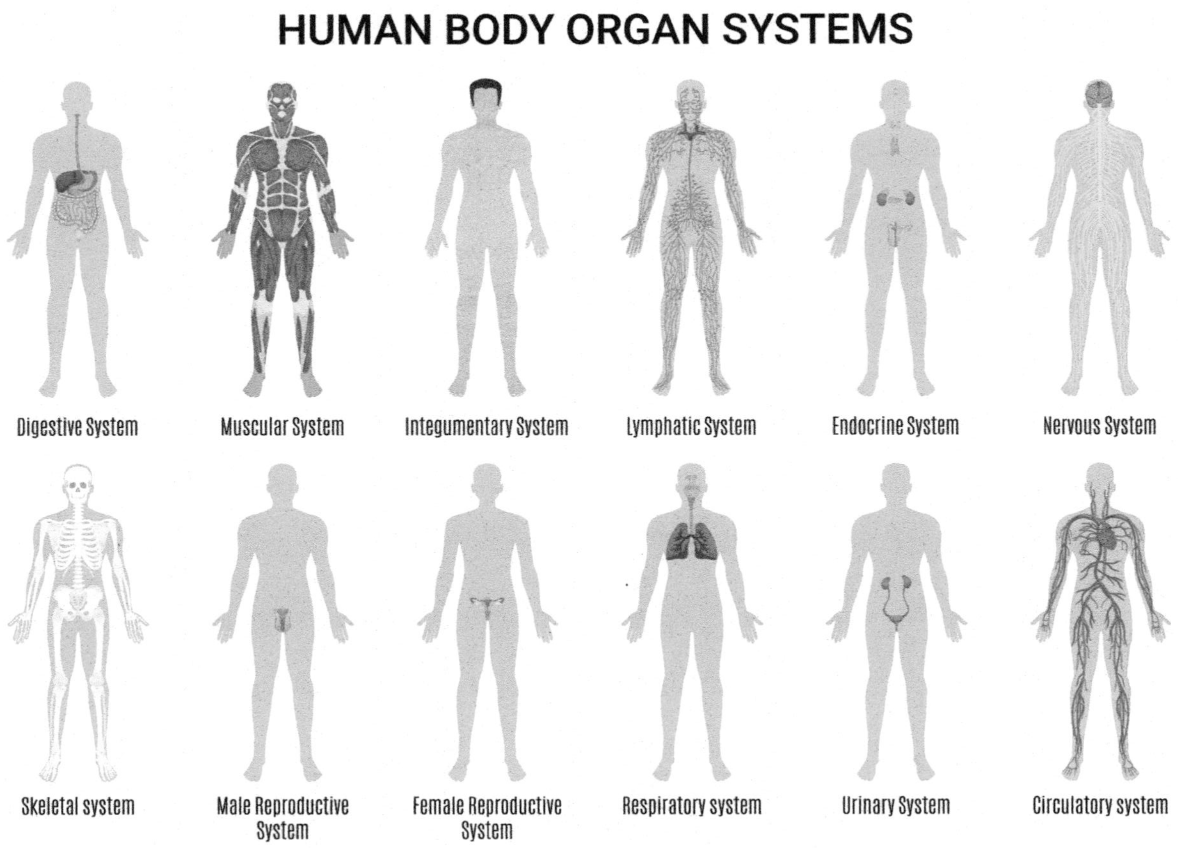

HUMAN BODY ORGAN SYSTEMS

Figure 1.1 Body organ systems.
Credit: macrovector/Shutterstock.com

III Dance nutrition vs sports nutrition

Dance nutrition has two main roles: to keep the body in the best of health possible and to 'support' the training program, so, eating for performance will ultimately change as the training regimen changes in terms of timing, quantity and source.

Nutrition advice for the dancer has many parallels to that for an athlete. The many similarities between sports and dance include, for instance, the development of technical abilities based on movement efficiency, the application of appropriate training regimens and concerns over injury prevention. Both athletes, and dancers train or perform almost every day, though dancers may well both train and perform; both may at times continue through pain (though this is not advisable), compete in challenging environments, experience little 'down time', face extreme competition and face a real risk of career-threatening injury. Comparing the work schedules of a professional performing artist and a professional baseball player highlights some of the similarities. Both perform/play in the evening (7 p.m. to 11 p.m. or later) with a schedule that may involve more than 150 games/performances a season. Dancers may well have more than one performance on several days of the week and can face challenges to fit in adequate food, particularly if nutrition is not prioritised as it needs to be. Changes to schedules can result in disturbed appetite and eating and sleeping habits. In this scenario, the professional sport athlete may well have access to nutrition information to help them understand what, why and when to eat, a team to provide support for injury prevention and rehab if needed, a biomechanist to address posture and movement patterns and a sport psychologist to optimise mental preparation and managing the workload. Currently, many dancers have few if any of these resources yet similar needs.

Both dance and sport require physical training. Although the actual training of the two will differ from each other for the most part, balance and agility are the most important skills to develop and hone in both. What can dance training offer the athlete? Training in dance can help athletes improve their flexibility, coordination and grace. Flexibility can allow athletes to use their full range of motion, which is beneficial in many sports, and may reduce the athlete's risk of injury. Coordination is very important in sports that require participants to be moving more than one part of your body at all times, which most sports do. Lastly, grace will help simply with the visual appeal of performance. From the other side, what can principles of sport science in training offer to the dancer? As with team sports, dance consists of intermittent sprint-type activity. Taking scientific principles from sport into dance will result in consideration of training sprint and endurance abilities, along with strength and stamina. Improving relevant aspects of fitness leaves the dancer free to focus on the artistic aspect of the dance in performance, rather than just achieving the sustained workload required in many performances whether musical theatre, ballet, contemporary, Irish or other genres.

There is an overlap between sport science and nutrition and dance science and nutrition where aesthetically judged sports, such as synchronised swimming and rhythmic gymnastics, have areas in common with dance. But dance is not always competitive; the focus is on art: the expression of human creative skill and imagination; performance conveys emotion which is not a feature in most sport.

Rodrigues-Krause et al. (2015) suggest that as dance had become more physically demanding, dance science has a key role and 'developing strategies to improve dancers' physical fitness should provide a foundation for optimising their artistic and technical skills. In essence, enhancing dancers' cardiorespiratory and neuromuscular systems would likely result in efficiency of movement, delayed fatigue onset and reduced susceptibility to injury'.

Sport nutrition is a fast-evolving area, as athletes from every sport seek to get the best from their performance. A summary by Professor Louise Burke (2021) reviewing the vast range of nutritional strategies that athletes use during competition events to optimise performance gives good insight into the current depth of the field of sports nutrition.

While dance nutrition draws from sports nutrition, it also considers that a dancer's goals and training and performance schedules are at least slightly different to those of an athlete, and dance nutrition research is the best evidence base for recommendations to dancers. There is a large gap still in this field and sufficient relevant high-quality information that can be translated into dance-specific guidelines and advice.

IV Dance fitness and nutrition

Dance fitness has a number of facets including strength, stamina, power, coordination and flexibility. Some dance styles require certain elements of fitness more explicitly than others, but dancers of all genres benefit from dance fitness. Nutrition plays a fundamental role in every area of dance fitness. A dance performance can require bursts of power but may also include extensive periods of movement of lower intensity in performances that may last for a few minutes (e.g. in a dance competition) or extend into multiple hours (e.g. Indian classical dance). Alongside this, nutrition requirements for dancers are not fixed: they vary across dance genres, from one dancer to another, depending on workload, during the training and performance seasons, and also vary in time away from dance such as holidays and, hopefully rarely, illness and injury. Nutrition is also an integral part of rest and recovery, where nutrients are required for the body to be at its best for the next period of dance.

Dance in general is characterised as an intermittent 'sprint' type of exercise, demanding energy from different metabolic pathways which are explored in Chapter 3. Intermittent exercise is characterised by a mixture of short sections of explosive moves and longer sections of lower-intensity movement. These have implications for metabolism because dancers attain high peaks of exercise intensity that alternate with active or passive recovery periods, where for oxygen consumption (VO_2) and heart rate (HR) are constantly changing, and with this energy use. It is recognised that dance performances take place at higher intensities than rehearsals or classes (Wyon et al., 2004) and nutrition intake needs to meet these higher demands or performance will suffer. The type of activity has an impact on the 'fuel' used: high-intensity work relies on carbohydrate, whereas both fats and carbohydrates will be used at lower intensities. The aim is not to use protein as a fuel, although this is a possibility if this is necessary. This will all be explored in detail in Chapters 3–6.

As with the variety between class, rehearsal and performance, there are also variations in the physical intensity, and thus fuel use, of classes. This can also vary from day to day and over a training or performance cycle, meaning that nutritional requirements also vary. As dancers become more expert in performing a movement or dance the energy demand will slightly reduce, meaning novices in any particular style and those facing new work need to be mindful of higher requirements until the work becomes more familiar. Dance genre also influences how a dancer trains and performs. Collegiate dancers in particularly have a unique challenge in balancing the dance term or semester, as this involves dance classes, rehearsals and performances alongside an academic responsibility and frequently there are financial challenges.

Understanding and working with all of these factors including primarily the need to periodise nutrition will allow the dancer to be optimally fuelled.

V Growth in the field of dance science: implications for nutrition

Dance science as an academic discipline is a relatively new and growing field: IADMS, the International Association of Dance Medicine and Science was founded in 1990 'with the goal to enhance the health, well-being, training and performance of dancers by cultivating medical, scientific and educational excellence while promoting an active network of communication between dance and medicine' (IADMS). It is the largest organisation promoting dance science internationally and allows the relatively small field of dance scientists globally to share best practice to support a population whose members themselves may not be training or working in their home country. The annual conference, which moves around the world, now sees nutrition presentations featuring consistently, while the peer-reviewed journal also features research on various aspects of dance nutrition.

The growth in dance science has translated into practical support for dancers. Individual countries may have dancer support organisations which incorporate dance science, such as the UK's OneDance UK, Ausdance in

Australia and Healthy Dancer Canada in Canada. These organisations will have a mission similar to that of OneDance UK, who state their goals as 'Our aim is to provide information, resources and opportunities for a workforce that is well-equipped to secure dance's prominence in the cultural landscape of the future' (OneDance UK). This will include information, or links to information, on dance science, including dance nutrition. There may be links to organisations such as the National Institute for Dance Medicine and Science (NIDMS) in the UK which was founded in 2012 to 'provide the dance sector with access to high quality, affordable, dance specific health care and dance science support services in private practice and the NHS' (NIDMS). Both IADMS and The Bridge Dance Project have a significant presence in the USA and can act as a conduit for disseminating information.

Degrees in Dance Science are becoming more widely available at both undergraduate and postgraduate levels. Nutrition is included in the curriculum with the overall aim of graduates having skills to apply scientific principles and evidence to dance. These skills can then be applied to support dancers to improve their health and well-being, enhance their performance and reduce their risk of injury.

Some vocational dance schools/colleges and dance companies employ dance scientists to provide input. This could include physiological testing, psychological support, strength and conditioning and nutritional input. As choreographic demands change, the benefits of these elements are increasingly valuable, and dancers not able to access input within their employment may find they benefit significantly by using directories to find qualified dance-specific practitioners. For nutrition, this can be via a registered dietitian or nutritionist who has dance expertise. Terminology for qualified practitioners will vary according to the country you are based in. A suitably expert practitioner will be able to consider each dancer as an individual and, in terms of nutrition, will consider the specific dance genre with current choreographic demands, schedules and workload together with travel and touring challenges if applicable.

Individual advice is needed for some dancers at some times. This book, the first comprehensive undergraduate nutrition book specifically for dancers, provides background and practical advice to get you started in assessing and reviewing your nutritional needs and changes that may benefit you. It can also guide you to identifying when you do need more specific individualised advice.

VI Resources

Sport Food Fact Sheet (bda.uk.com).
Factsheets Archive – Sports Dietitians Australia (SDA).
Nutrition (teamusa.org).
Home|Mysportscience a trusted source of information.

VII Learning outcomes

After reading this chapter the reader should be able to:

1   Explain how nutrition can support the dancer to perform at their best.
2   Discuss the growth in the field of Dance Science over the last 30 years.

References

Burke, L.M. (2021) Nutritional approaches to counter performance constraints in high-level sports competition, *Experimental Physiology*, 106(12), pp.2304–2323.
Rodrigues-Krause, J., Krause, M. and Reischak-Oliveira, Á. (2015) Cardiorespiratory considerations in dance: From classes to performances, *Journal of Dance Medicine & Science*, 19(3), pp.91–102.
Wyon, M.A. et al. (2004) Oxygen uptake during modern dance class, rehearsal, and performance, *The Journal of Strength & Conditioning Research*, 18(3), pp.646–649.

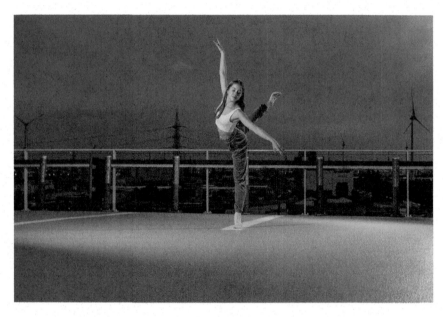

Photo 2.1 Identifying and prioritising nutrition goals and strategies will pay off in the studio and in performance.

Source: Photo courtesy of Robert Biesemans.

2   Food and the dancer

Contents

I Nutrition: a priority for dancers?

Dancers demand a lot of their bodies. They become accustomed to pushing their bodies to the limit. Performing at a high level is expected from early in training, particularly for those looking to dance professionally. Everyone has the ability to dance and to enjoy dance, but performing complex and intricately beautiful movement to a professional level is a talent not possessed by many. Translating potential into reality requires extensive time, energy and focus. During training and a professional career, dancers experience many physiological and psychological challenges including injuries. The dancer's experience of life can be significantly impacted if their body's ability to function becomes compromised. For a dancer to understand their body and its particular needs requires reflection and patience and recognition of changes that occur over time. In terms of nutritional needs, dancers are best supported when the team supporting them, whether this is in training or at work, understand and address, as far as practical, the challenges dancers face in meeting their nutritional needs. These challenges include having sufficient knowledge to make appropriate decisions for the current situation; time pressures; access to food; enough energy – both physical and psychological – to plan and implement a suitable meal plan; travel commitments and financial concerns.

DOI: 10.4324/9781003219002-2

Dancers are used to taking note of how movement feels in their body but may have become less familiar with taking note of the feedback they receive from the systems related to nutritional intake. Dance training schedules in particular can take inadequate note of the basic human – including dancer humans – need for fuel to carry out the work required. Over-running classes and rehearsals are common and can leave dancers challenged to take on board appropriate nutrition and fluid. In addition, for the dancer to be able to appropriately prioritise, this need for fuel and hydration requires them to have a healthy relationship with their body and be able to thoughtfully process the huge amount of feedback from the body to the brain, as well as the responses from the brain to the body. There may well be some compromises required; the challenge is to keep these to levels which don't compromise health, well-being or performance. Healthy levels of self-esteem are likely to be behind dancers who are able to appropriately provide their body with appropriate food and fluids in the face of situations where the end product is valued above the dancers' well-being.

Dance as an art form is an umbrella under which there are a wide variety of genres, which continue to evolve and some of which are becoming difficult to categorise because they are influenced by two or more styles. These include, singly or merged, ballet, modern, contemporary, jazz, tap, hip-hop, street, breaking, ballroom, musical theatre, plus those more specific to a country or population such as Indian, Irish, Spanish, Scottish and African. As yet dance nutrition research is focussed on a narrow range of these genres, and cross-genre take-home messages need careful consideration. And of course most dancers in training and also professionals regularly engage in several genres. Ballet is the most researched form of dance overall, but numbers of studies in dance are a fraction of those in sport, meaning that frequently it is necessary to look at research on comparable activities with regard to exercise intensity and adapt information to support best practice in dance. There is a research focus on injury management and prevention in dance, although injury prevention is now more frequently being looked at as injury risk reduction. This acknowledges that some level of injury is unfortunately unavoidable, but there are many causes which can be mitigated. Russell (2013) in a review entitled 'Preventing dance injuries: current perspectives' identified five essential components for those involved with caring for dancers that, when properly applied, will assist them in decreasing the likelihood of dance-related injury and ensuring that dancers receive optimum attention from the health care profession: (1) screening; (2) physical training; (3) nutrition and rest; (4) specialised dance health care; and (5) becoming acquainted with the nature of dance and dancers.

II Body image in dance

The dancer's unique relationship with their body: the role of body image

The expectation for dancers in some genres, ballet in particular, over recent decades, has been that they will be slim, or even thin, well-proportioned and toned. Some have been put under a great deal of pressure to maintain a body with very low body fat levels, while others struggle with the belief that they needs to be smaller than they are (Kalyva et al., 2021). This has been recognised as contributing to disordered eating and eating disorders (Polivy & Herman, 2004). There are various aspects of the dance class that can potentially lead to a negative body image, including language used. Body image can be defined as the combination of thoughts and feelings that a dancer has about their body. This can include both negative and positive thoughts and feelings and is impacted by both external and internal factors. Body image concerns are known to start at a young age: they can start in young children, whether or not they are dancers, before they reach puberty (Hughes et al., 2018). Puberty, with the changes that occur, is a time when dancers in training benefit from particular support to weather the challenges of managing a body that has changing proportions and where movement will be different to how it was previously, whether due to longer limbs, or differences in growth rates of muscles, bones and tendons.

A positive body image is hard to sustain in a critical environment, which dance can be but protects against eating disorders and is the goal. Perhaps the first step is for dancers in training to be supported to have at least a neutral body image, in other words body acceptance: the ability to accept their body even when not feeling positive about all of it, in order to be able to meet their nutritional needs. There are a number of strategies that have been trialled for improving body image that can make a difference and these are summarised in Table 2.1 (adapted from Alleva et al., 2015). Although most will need input from a suitably qualified psychologist or therapist, it is helpful to know that body image is not fixed, and negative body image can be improved. Some techniques were shown to be unhelpful, including

Table 2.1 Strategies known to improve body image

Strategies that improve body image

Changing negative body language: This technique directly targets the language that people use to describe or talk about their body, with the aim of helping individuals to use objective or positive terms rather than negative, judgmental language and avoiding comments or conversations that are focussed on weight and appearance.

Psychoeducation: Learning about and understanding about what can influence body image can give people a better understanding of the factors that precipitate and exacerbate negative body image, and may help them to recognise and manage the impact of 'triggers' (e.g., media, social media showing idealised bodies).

Guided imagery: Visualising accepting the body – guided by a therapist/psychologist.

Exposure exercises: Challenging a fear, supported by a therapist/psychologist.

Size-estimate exercises: Challenging the inaccurate perception of body size, supported by a psychologist/therapist.

---

discussing physical fitness and discussing individual differences. Ensuring that conversations do not focus on weight and appearance is a strategy that can usefully be used in every aspect of a dancer's life.

Having a negative body image can lead dancers to turn to their diet as a means to try and change their body. Dieting is a risk factor for eating disorders and disordered eating, which can in turn have a major impact on quality of life and may interfere with training or work plans for dancers.

There are some aspects of the dancer's life that may additionally impact on body image, for example mirrors: some studios have mirrors, whereas others don't. Anecdotally almost every mirror has areas which do not accurately reflect body size, having either a magnifying or a shrinking effect – like a subtle hall of mirrors. To work next to a mirror that is distorting body shape in the reflection is a challenge to body image, although there appears to be a lack of research on this topic. Partner and group work with lifts is another aspect that impacts on few students or working adults outside dance, circus and team acrobatic/cheerleading. While the experience can be very positive, this is dependent on the language and approach used. Any experiences that result in a dancer believing they need to be smaller are likely to impact on nutrition choices and intake.

III Unintentional underfuelling: RED-S

The workload for a dancer in training can typically be based on dance or other physical activity for 4½ hours or more on at least five days per week during an academic term or semester. When assessments or performances – or both – are looming this workload can increase, so the working day may start before 9 a.m. in the morning and continue with rehearsal or performances until late in the evening. There may be gaps, but some students may be dancing for up to ten hours or more per day at points in the year. The situation is not necessarily easier for professionals. Research with professional ballet dancers found they were active for eight hours at work plus additional time outside their work schedule (Kozai et al., 2020). This workload can make it difficult to find the time and energy to consistently plan, shop for, prepare and eat adequate meals and snacks. Dancers when short of time during the day may not eat enough, and if tired in the evening may opt for a snack rather than a meal and can end up unintentionally underfuelled, experiencing what has been termed relative energy deficiency in sport (RED-S). This condition, which includes the better known female athlete triad but applies to all athletes and dancers, was first described in 2014 and is explored in detail in Chapter 11. It is important for dancers to be aware of and avoid or resolve as quickly as possible, as the impact is on most body systems and can impact performance. RED-S can also occur where the energy deficiency is precipitated by disordered eating or an eating disorder, in which case the dancer will primarily need support for the disordered eating. Once this has hopefully resolved the dancer may well be able to meet their energy needs and avoid energy deficiency.

There is already evidence that dancers are experiencing RED-S, with a study of female ballet students which found energy expenditure exceeded reported intake, low body weight and hormonal disturbances (Civil et al., 2019). A study using an online questionnaire also found that over 25% of the dancers, both male and female, who responded, were experiencing physical, physiological and psychological changes consistent with low energy availability and were at risk of RED-S (Keay et al., 2020). Although there was a major campaign in 2019 to target athletes at risk of RED-S, using the name '#trainbrave', this did not reach dancers, and awareness of RED-S is growing more slowly.

IV Nutrition and injury

There are several thousand research papers on injury in dancers, indicating that this is a topic of interest. This is unlikely to be a surprise to any dancer of probably every genre: perhaps there are dance genres where injuries are not experienced, but it seems unlikely. There are some areas of the body known to be more at risk of becoming injured than others, for example foot and ankle injuries rather than hand or arm injuries, but because injuries can occur for a number of reasons, including those outside the dancer's control, any part of the body can be injured in dance, even if the risk for some body parts is incredibly low. Both anecdotally and from research evidence most dance students will experience at least one injury per year (Nordin-Bates et al., 2011). Professional dancers also experience injuries, which are most frequently identified as due to overuse, with one systematic review of reported injury studies on ballet injuries finding a frequency of 2.8 injuries per dancer over the reporting time periods, which was a maximum of one year (Smith et al., 2016).

The links between nutrition and injury

When nutritional intake isn't enough to meet requirements, the dancer is likely to fatigue more easily and also to have less good focus and concentration than if they have an adequate intake of either or both water and nutrients. Both fatigue and reduced focus can increase the risk of injury, and this may be greater when undertaking repetitive activity. Although dancers tend to have a higher pain threshold than non-dancers (Russell, 2013), many dancers do regularly experience pain, and this in itself can impact both on appetite and on motivation and ability to meet their nutritional requirements. Dancers who have joint hypermobility syndrome (JHS) may suffer more with pain from their digestive system as there is a link between JHS and functional gastrointestinal symptoms, including IBS (Fragkos et al., 2019). IBS is discussed further in Chapter 13.

V Challenges to dancers' nutrition

Dancers face a number of challenges to nutrition in addition to the areas already explored. These areas are reviewed now, with some practical recommendations to minimise the impact as far as is possible.

1   *Skills for self-catering*

While it is possible to survive and get all the nutrients needed from cold food, this can rapidly become uninspiring and requires knowledge and planning to make sure no nutrients get missed. Some dancers become adept at preparing nutrient-dense meals and snacks by their mid-teens, others may still have limited skills several years later. Dancers looking at self-catering for the first time will benefit from acquiring the skills to be able to plan and prepare a range of suitable meals that will meet daily requirements in advance of the change. This requires the knowledge of what is required nutritionally to fuel dance and the practical skills to cook at least a basic minimum range of meals.

If at all possible any student who will need to cook some, or all, of their own meals is advised to arrive at the start of their first term/ semester with the knowledge and skills to prepare a week's worth of main meals. This doesn't necessarily mean seven completely different meals, although this would be a good starting point. Repeating a meal twice in one week where that meal includes good quality protein (information on this in Chapter 5), at least two different vegetables, and some carbohydrate puts the dancer more at risk of boredom from the repetition more than any concerns over nutritional adequacy, if the other meals are varied. Practical understanding of cooking terms will facilitate exploration of new recipes and broadening the range of foods eaten. Dancers who are moving from one country to another can face challenges in finding familiar foods and can benefit from support, if possible, while they settle in. Some dancers are confident cooks and relish the opportunity to explore new foods, but this is not the case for all. For sure experience makes a huge difference in cooking main meals, but some dancers will have no option but to learn while settling into full-time training.

2   *Time*

Time to plan, shop for, cook and eat adequately can be a challenge. Dancers are rarely in control of their schedule, which in any case may be prone to change at short notice. Meal prepping, preparing meals for several days in bulk at one time to be frozen and/or kept in the fridge, is a great strategy but does require planning and finding enough time to do, most likely on a non-dance day.

3   *Access to food*

Whether as a student based in a remote location, as a professional dancer on tour, or when a schedule runs across planned meal breaks, there can be times when access to food is less than optimal. Each of these situations, and others where food access is limited, can have an impact on nutrition. There will generally be a solution, but this may not be obvious until too late. Approaching any new situation, fact finding is rarely a waste of time and can minimise the chances of the unhelpful unexpected situation.

4 *Financial challenges*

Many dancers, whether students or professionals, have a limited food budget. For some, the budget may be tight but is sufficient to meet all nutrient needs. This is likely to mean opting for cheaper sources of protein, in particular, thinking carefully before buying drinks or snacks while away from home, making rather than buying snack items where possible and opting for the lower prices sources of carbs and fats. Food can still be enjoyable, but it will be more of a challenge than when there is more money available for food. For others, the amount of money that can be made available for food is not enough, whether temporarily or longer term. This situation is not compatible with either training or performance, and any dancer in this position will struggle to continue to dance. Students are best to speak with their training institution, as help is often available for those in real need. Professional dancers facing food insecurity are in an incredibly difficult position, to which there is no obvious or easy solution. In the short term, using food banks and apps such as 'Too Good To Go' and 'OLIO' can be helpful, but for the longer term, it will be necessary to find a solution that can, if at all possible, provide an income that includes adequate money for nutrition.

5 *Knowledge*

Before thinking about improving knowledge, dancers need to be aware of the role that nutrition plays in their health, well-being and ability to dance throughout their career. For a dancer to spend time identifying their own individual challenges is worthwhile: this is necessary to generate their own individual solution in conjunction with relevant information and resources. They can then work on improving their knowledge of nutrition for dancer training and performance. This book is a good place to start.

VI Dancer nutrition goals

Dancers will benefit from recognising that nutrition is an important tool in their training programme and performance support strategies. Understanding the need for adequate amounts of both macro and micronutrients, and how to meet their own needs will allow energy, growth and repair systems to work optimally – in conjunction with appropriate dance and rest schedules. This book aims to provide a comprehensive review of nutrition for dancers, with sufficient detail to allow those who wish to calculate quantities of nutrients which then will be translated into food portions for their requirements.

Table 2.2 Dancer nutrition goals

Nutrition goals for the dancer
To be adequately hydrated and have good energy stores before starting class/rehearsal/performance
To use food and fluids to optimise recovery after dance or other activity
To meet daily nutritional requirements for all macronutrients including omega 3 fatty acids, as well as vitamins, minerals, using appropriate supplements if needed
To include adequate plant-based foods to benefit from phytochemicals
To incorporate any changes for special diet followed for medical or other reasons without compromising nutritional intake

Others will opt to avoid calculations and go for the qualitative information, which should again guide the dancer to meeting requirements, even as these vary from day to day and week to week. Table 2.2 summarises the roles of nutrition in aspects of the dancer's life that will benefit the dancer to be curious about and explore where and how any changes needed can best be made.

The next chapters tackle the macronutrients dancers require and then move onto more applied topics. Each chapter stands alone, though does include links to other chapters where information sits between two or more areas.

VII Resources

Burke, L.M., Castell, L.M., Casa, D.J., Close, G.L., Costa, R.J., Desbrow, B., Halson, S.L., Lis, D.M., Melin, A.K., Peeling, P. and Saunders, P.U., 2019. International association of athletics federations consensus statement 2019: Nutrition for athletics. *International Journal of Sport Nutrition and Exercise Metabolism*, 29(2), pp. 73–84.
https://www.bda.uk.com/resource/food-facts-eat-well-spend-less.html.
https://www.nutrition.gov/topics/shopping-cooking-and-meal-planning/food-shopping-and-meal-planning.

VIII Learning outcomes

At the end of this chapter the reader should be able to:

1   Identify nutritional goals for dancers.
2   List at least four reasons why dancers' may struggle to meet their nutritional requirements.
3   Describe the links between nutrition and injury.

References

Alleva, J.M. et al. (2015) A meta-analytic review of stand-alone interventions to improve body image, *PLoS One*, 10(9), pe0139177.

Civil, R. et al. (2019) Assessment of dietary intake, energy status, and factors associated with RED-S in vocational female ballet students, *Frontiers in Nutrition*, 5, pp.136.

Fragkos, K.C. et al. (2019) Joint hypermobility syndrome affects response to a low fermentable oligosaccharide, disaccharide, monosaccharide and polyol diet in irritable bowel syndrome patients: A retrospective study, *Gastroenterology Research*, 12(1), p.27.

Hughes, E.K. et al. (2018) Body image dissatisfaction and the adrenarchal transition, *Journal of Adolescent Health,* 63(5), pp.621–627.

Kalyva, S. et al. (2021) Disturbed eating attitudes, social physique anxiety, and perceived pressure for thin body in professional dancers, *Research in Dance Education*, 6(12), pp.1–12.

Keay, N., Overseas, A. and Francis, G. (2020) Indicators and correlates of low energy availability in male and female dancers, *BMJ Open Sport & Exercise Medicine*, 6(1), pp.e000906.

Kozai, A.C. et al. (2020) Workload intensity and rest periods in professional ballet: Connotations for injury, *International Journal of Sports Medicine*, 41(06), pp.373–379.

Nordin-Bates, S.M. et al. (2011) Injury, imagery, and self-esteem in dance healthy minds in injured bodies? *Journal of Dance Medicine & Science*, 15(2), pp.76–85.

Polivy, J. and Herman, C.P. (2004) Sociocultural idealization of thin female body shapes: An introduction to the special issue on body image and eating disorders, *Journal of Social and Clinical Psychology*, 23(1), pp.1–6.

Russell, J.A. (2013) Preventing dance injuries: Current perspectives, *Open Access Journal of Sports Medicine*, 4, pp.199.

Smith, T.O. et al. (2016) Prevalence and profile of musculoskeletal injuries in ballet dancers: A systematic review and meta-analysis, *Physical Therapy in Sport*, 19, pp.50–56.

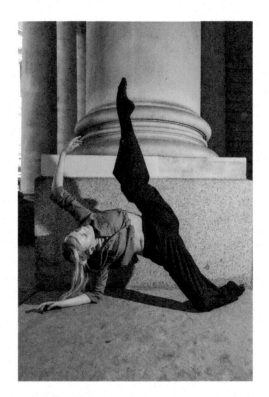

Photo 3.1 The human body switches seamlessly between energy systems which allows dancers to focus on performance.
Source: Photo courtesy of Mike Cooper.

3   Energy for dance

Contents

I Introduction

Metabolism can be considered as 'the chemical processes that occur within a living organism to maintain life'.

From the time you eat and drink food or fluids, that supply nutrients, it takes typically several hours before these foods and fluids are processed ready for the cells of your body to use. First, foods, which have an initial huge variety of structures and contents, must be broken down into their basic components during digestion, then the nutrients need to be absorbed into the blood stream to then finally reach their destination in the body, for example, the muscle fibres (muscle cells) in the legs or arms. The digestive system will be explored in more detail shortly. The main part of the digestive system – effectively a tube that runs from the stomach through the small intestine (SI) to the large intestine (LI) – is usually known as the gut, and this shorthand term will be used in this and subsequent chapters.

DOI: 10.4324/9781003219002-3

Foods contain many different nutrients; there are also components of food that are not of use. The two main categories of nutrients are macronutrients and micronutrients. Macronutrients are explored in this chapter. Micronutrients are vitamins and minerals, which are needed by the body in very small amounts, typically under 1 g/day, and which have many and varied roles, including enabling energy to be released from macronutrients. They are explored in Appendix A.

II Macronutrients: the nutrients involved in energy production

Energy is needed for life processes as well as activity

Macronutrient is the term for those nutrients which humans – including dancers – consume in significant quantities; daily intakes are measured in grams. Water, essential for hydration, is sometimes considered a macronutrient but does not supply energy so is being considered separately in Chapter 7. Macronutrients can be metabolised by the body to produce energy to fuel the basic requirements of the body – including maintaining heartbeat, core temperature, lung function and fuelling the brain – and activity, such as dance.

At a cellular level in your body, the fuel used is adenosine triphosphate (ATP). Macronutrients are used to maintain levels of ATP. At any given time, there is only enough ATP stored for one to two seconds of maximal effort exercise; after this, stores need to be replaced by metabolising macronutrients.

What are the macronutrients?

There are three main macronutrients: carbohydrates (carbs), fats and protein. Alcohol is technically a macronutrient and does provide energy but will only be considered very briefly as the effects on the nervous system make it unsuitable as a fuel for activity. Although protein can be used as a fuel, protein is unique in being needed for repair and growth of muscle, tendons, ligaments, skin and bone. Protein also has a role in many other essential body functions as well as generally being more expensive both in price and to the environment. This will be explored further in Chapter 5. Because protein is needed for many roles in the body that no other nutrient can fulfil, dancers are advised to focus on taking in adequate carbohydrates and fats for energy rather than relying on protein as an energy source. The roles of carbs, fats and protein are introduced in this chapter before each is explored in more detail in the following chapters.

Measuring energy content in food

Foods can be analysed to determine the amount of each macronutrient as well as the energy content they contain. This energy available from food from macronutrients is measured in either kilocalories, abbreviated to kcal or kilojoules, abbreviated to kJ. The amount of fibre and other components, particularly in plant-based foods, can slightly reduce the availability of macro-nutrients and energy in practice, but there is currently a lack of data on this.

How are macronutrients used in the cell?

Once the nutrients have entered the cells of the body there are a number of steps that take place first in the cytosol and more particularly in the mito-chondria of those cells. The Krebs cycle (also known as the citric acid cycle, or the TCA cycle) is a major part of this, a complex pathway in the mito-chondria where the energy-supplying nutrients are metabolised. Carbohy-drates and fatty acids enter Krebs cycle after being converted into Acetyl CoA. This release of energy from the chemical bonds in food is added to the body stores of ATP. As mentioned above, ATP is the store for energy in every cell. Carbon dioxide is produced in this process. The carbon dioxide

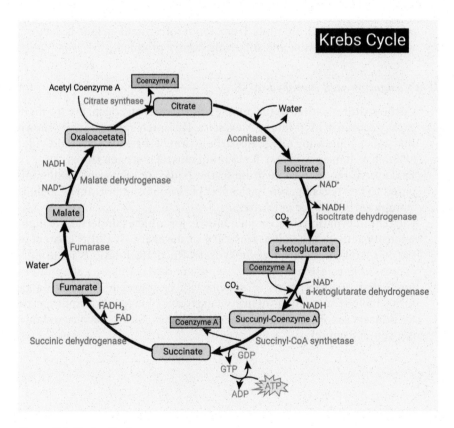

Figure 3.1 Krebs Cycle.
Credit: Jo Sam Re/Shutterstock.com

will be transported back to the lungs and then breathed out. A form of nicotinamide adenine dinucleotide (NADH) produced during the Krebs cycle will be used in other essential reaction within the body (Figure 3.1).

III Introduction to carbohydrate structure and function

Carbohydrate structures

- Carbohydrates are made from carbon, hydrogen, and oxygen, with two atoms of each of carbon and oxygen for every atom of hydrogen, for example glucose and fructose have the same composition $C_6H_{12}O_6$, although they do have different structures which result in fructose being significantly sweeter than glucose.
- Carbohydrates are synthesised by plants which form sugars and starches (longer molecules than sugars).
- Glycogen, the human storage form of carbohydrate, is structurally like starch. For vegans and those dancers not including dairy, the carbohydrate in their diet is exclusively plant based: the only carbohydrate available in useful amounts from foods of animal origin is lactose, which is found in milk and some other dairy products.

Why do dancers need carbohydrates?

- Carbohydrates, stored in the muscles and liver as glycogen, are the main energy source in high-intensity exercise. Research has repeatedly shown that a diet containing adequate carbohydrate is best for active individuals such as dancers. This will maintain muscle glycogen stores.
- Because stores of carbohydrate in the body are relatively small compared to fat stores in even the leanest person, it is important to include enough carbohydrate in the diet.
- Current international recommendations for athletes undertaking high-intensity activity are that at least 50% of the energy (calorie) content of the diet should come from carbohydrate. Recommendations are usually expressed in g carb per kg body weight per day as this way adaptations for higher or lower levels of activity can be covered. As most dance forms include some high-intensity (anaerobic) activity, it is appropriate for dancers to follow the guidelines for athletes. More specific guidance is given in Chapter 4.

Nutritional benefits of carb-rich foods

Food type	Additional nutrients provided	Note
Fruits	Vitamin C, phytochemicals, potassium, vitamin A, folate	For more information on the vital role vitamins and minerals play in health and performance go to Appendix A
Grains and products made from them, e.g. bread, pasta, couscous, noodles	Protein, iron, B vitamins	
Starchy vegetables	Vitamin A (sweet potato), vitamin C and potassium (potatoes)	

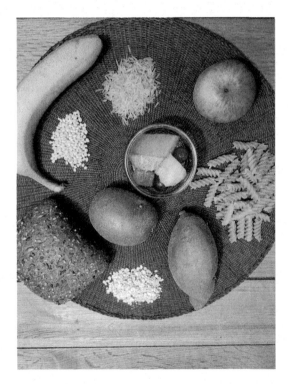

Photo 3.2 Carb-rich foods.

How much energy does carbohydrate supply, and how quickly is it available?

- For reference, carbohydrates supply 3.75 kcal/g. For labelling purposes, this is rounded up to 4 kcal/g (16 kJ/g). Carbohydrates can be found in both minimally and highly processed foods.
- Both the type of food and the other nutrients it contains impact on the speed the carbohydrates are digested and thus made available to the body. When carbohydrates are digested, they impact on the blood glucose levels in the body.
- Foods from which the carbohydrates are available quickly and impact rapidly on blood glucose levels are known as high glycaemic index foods, while those where the carbohydrate digestion and absorption are slower are referred to as low glycaemic index foods.

Do all carbohydrates have the same effects in the body?

- Both low and high glycaemic index foods can have a role in fuelling the dancer. Low glycaemic index foods are useful if eaten some time before dance, for less rapid energy release, whereas high glycaemic index foods have a role when time is short during training and they allow re-fuelling to start quickly after performance.
- Consuming high glycaemic index foods during activity doesn't seem to cause swings in blood sugar levels that are often seen at rest (Oosthuyse et al., 2015), and these foods are likely to be easier to digest.
- Because they are often less rich in other nutrients it is important you think about the balance of different carbs in your diet. This will be looked at further in Chapter 4.
- There is evidence that depending on the level of processing not all the energy is available to be used by the body: Dr Giles Yeo is promoting this work (New Scientist 16/6/2021) but in 2022 food labelling still provides information assuming 100% of the energy is available.

Fibre is categorised as a carbohydrate, how is it different to other carbs?

Fibre is the part of food not digested in the SI. Some types of fibre will be metabolised by gut bacteria with the production of fatty acids which are available to the body, whereas other fibres pass through the digestive system unaltered.
   Different compositions have different effects:

- Some types, often known as insoluble, are important to prevent constipation.
- Some types, known as soluble, help to regulate blood sugar levels.
- More soluble fibre is found in oats, fruit and pulses [lentils and beans] and more insoluble is found in wholegrain products.

Practical advice: fibre for dancers

If you are following fruit and vegetable guidelines of 5+ servings per day, including wholegrain foods where possible, for example wholemeal bread, brown rice and including pulses and oats regularly, then you will have an adequate fibre intake. Some dancers, for example those with digestive problems, may in fact need to reduce their fibre intake. This is very individual and will be looked at in more detail in Chapter 13.

IV Introduction to fat structure and function

Structure

- Fats, like carbohydrates, are made up of carbon, hydrogen and oxygen, but the ratio is different, and this has a major impact on both the consistency of fats and how they are metabolised, which is particularly relevant during exercise (Figure 3.2).

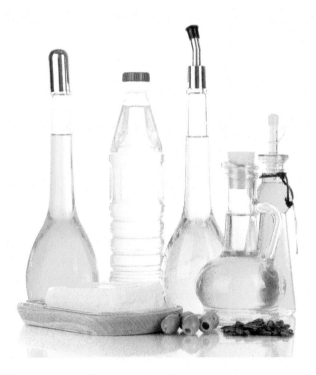

Figure 3.2 Plant sources of fat tend to liquid at room temperature, animal sources tend to be solid.
Credit: Africa Studio/Shutterstock.com

- Fats in foods consist of three fatty acids joined to a glycerol (chemical formula C3H8O3) molecule. Typically, fatty acids contain 12–18 atoms of carbon, though some may have as few as four or as many as 36.
- There are three types of fat, according to the chemical structure: saturated, monounsaturated and polyunsaturated. The common structure of all fats is that they have chains of carbon and hydrogen atoms, which have a carboxyl group – COOH – on the end.
- Saturated fats have all possible positions filled with hydrogen atoms, while unsaturated do not.
- Monounsaturated have just one position where further hydrogen could be added.
- The differing structures lead to different properties – unsaturated fats tend to be liquid at room temperature, e.g. vegetable oils, whereas saturated fats tend to be of animal origin and be solid at room temperature – butter, lard and meat fat.

Function

- Regardless of the structure fats supply 9 kcal or 37 kJ/gram, and so are a much more concentrated source of energy than carbohydrates.
- It is useful to remember that as well as supplying energy, fats are necessary to allow some vitamins, those which are fat soluble, to be absorbed. For more information on this and of the role of these vitamins in dancer health, see Appendix A.
- Saturated fats are linked with heart disease, although there is discussion as to whether this is all saturated fats, e.g. dairy versus pastry.
- Unsaturated fats – mono- and polyunsaturated such as olive oil the fat in nuts and seeds (mono), sunflower oil and fish oils (poly) tend to protect against heart disease, if taken in the recommended amounts.

Requirements

The aim should be to include sufficient energy from fat in the diet to meet energy requirements. The typical UK/US diet contains 35–36% energy from fat. The recommendation for athletes – and dancers – is to consume 20–30% of the calories in the food from fat (Thomas et al., 2016). This should result in an intake between 40 and 90 g/day depending on energy requirements. Aiming for around 1 g fat per kg body weight is generally a good starting point; this will be explored from a practical perspective in Chapter 6.

Requirements for specific fats

Essential fatty acids (EFA) are a subgroup of polyunsaturated fats

EFA are seen as essential because you must consume them from foods, rather than being able to adapt another substance to make them yourself. They can supply energy to the body, but have crucial roles in health. Although for many years it wasn't clear of the role of EFA in adults, it was well known that EFA are essential for brain development in children. It is now recognised that EFA have a role in many functions in the body, including eyesight, brain function, metabolism, inflammation, our immune system, wound healing, blood clotting and the proper functioning of the liver, kidneys, heart and muscles.

EFA come from two sources:

Omega-3 from alpha-linolenic acid particularly from oily fish, linseeds, pumpkin seeds, walnuts, rapeseed oil and fortified soybeans.

Omega-6 from linoleic acid particularly from vegetable oils.

Omega-3 fatty acids may enhance aerobic metabolism.

EFA will be explored further in Chapter 6.

Differences between carbs and fats

Nutrient	Chemical composition	When are they useful?	Examples of foods with a high content of the nutrient
Carbohydrates (carbs)	Carbon, hydrogen and oxygen, e.g. glucose $C_6H_{12}O_6$	Used for energy, particularly for high-intensity activity	Grains and foods made from grains such as oats, pasta, maize, bread, rice, quinoa, (sweet) potatoes, fruit

Introduction to protein structure and function

Protein structure

- Protein molecules are made up of building blocks called amino acids, which contain carbon, hydrogen and oxygen with the addition of nitrogen, and in some cases, sulphur.
- Amino acids link together into peptide chains via chemical bonds, known as peptide bonds, to make up peptides and proteins. Peptides contain between 2 and about 50 amino acids joined together, whereas proteins contain over 50 amino acids joined together.
- Amino acids have a central carbon atom, a hydrogen atom, a carboxyl group (COOH), an amino group (NH_2) and a side chain. The impact of different side chains is discussed in Chapter 5.

- When protein in food is digested it is broken down into peptides and then into amino acids before being rebuilt into the proteins needed by the body, for example in muscle, skin, ligaments and tendons.
- There are 21 amino acids, 9 of which are described as 'essential amino acids' (EAA) or 'indispensable amino acids'. These are confusing terms as in fact you need all 21 amino acids – but you cannot synthesise EAA – they must be obtained from food.
- Some amino acids have been identified as conditionally essential/ indispensable where they become essential in specific situations such as when the body has experienced stress. This group includes six amino acids, and more research is needed to clarify when each may become essential. The remaining six amino acids can be synthesised within the body.

Protein functions

- Protein is needed for many purposes including the formation of enzymes which are essential for many body processes to take place and for antibodies a crucial part of your immune system as well as being essential for the well-known functions of growth and repair. This is looked at in more detail in Chapter 5.
- One additional purpose that is related to energy supplies within the body is as part of the energy supply system: creatine phosphate is synthesised from glycine in the liver, and two additional amino acids, arginine and methionine are involved in the process. Creatine phosphate, also known as phosphocreatine, can provide energy for about five to eight seconds of maximal exertion, after which stores need to be replaced. This is discussed further below.
- Protein in the body is constantly being broken down and created. Daily protein turnover is around 4 g/kg bodyweight per day, which is several times more than your daily intake (Lanham-New et al., 2019).
- As a macronutrient protein can be used as an energy source, and this will happen if excess protein is consumed. If protein is used for energy, it will provide 4 kcal/g.
- Current recommendations of the levels of protein which are needed for optimum performance in highly active individuals are however well above the recommendations for the general populations, and dancers are more at risk of not taking in enough protein than excess.
- If excess protein is consumed, then it can either be used for energy immediately, or it can be stored as fat. Overfeeding protein results in a greater amount of energy being transformed into heat than for either fat or carbohydrate, and energy stored will be less than predicted if this is not considered (Lanham-New et al., 2019).

There is a situation however where protein is used as a source of fuel because a dancer is not taking in enough energy in total. In this circumstance, protein can be metabolised for energy and additionally fat and potentially muscle are broken down to meet the energy deficit. Higher protein intakes have been shown to prevent muscle breakdown even when energy is limited, in short-term studies, if resistance exercise is undertaken (Pasiakos et al., 2014). It is important to be aware that not all dancers under-fuelling will experience the extensive negative physical consequences seen in relative energy deficiency in sport (RED-S) (see Chapter 11).

Protein-rich foods supply micronutrients

Foods rich in protein typically also provide good sources of one or more micronutrients in the diet. For example, red meat and dark chicken meat are good sources of iron and vitamin B12, white fish is a good source of iodine, eggs are a good source of selenium, vitamins D and B12 and tofu is a good source of calcium.

Introduction to energy use during exercise

Fat is the main fuel used in low-intensity long duration exercise. The mechanism regulating which fuel the body chooses is not well understood. If there is a lack of both carbohydrate and fat, then protein either from food or from muscle may be used. What is well understood is that as exercise intensity increases, the body becomes more reliant on carbohydrate stores and fat use reduces. If exercise continues beyond 30 minutes, the muscles gradually begin to rely less on muscle glycogen and muscle triglycerides and more on plasma free fatty acids for their energy.

Exercise intensity is often expressed as a percentage of VO_2 Max. As you exercise with increasing intensity, the amount of oxygen you breathe in and process increases up to your maximum, your VO_2 Max, usually measured usually in litres per minute. Although exercise intensity may continue to increase, there comes a point where you can no longer increase how much oxygen you can process and deliver to the body, and you have to produce energy from nutrients without oxygen. This is discussed in more detail shortly. VO_2 Max is usually expressed relative to body weight: ml/minute/kg body weight. See Table 3.1 for information on how the use of each energy source changes with increasing exercise intensity.

In Table 3.1, please note that energy used is in calories not kcal.

Table 3.1 Contribution of different energy sources as exercise intensity increases

Source of energy in exercise	Approximate amount of energy at 30 minutes exercise (cal/kg/min) at increasing %VO_2 Max		
	25%VO_2 Max	65%VO_2 Max	85%VO_2 Max
Muscle glycogen	negligible	80	165
Muscle triglycerides	10	50	35
Plasma glucose	10	20	35
Plasma free fatty acids	65	55	40

Source: Based on data including that from Romijn et al. (1993).

The 'fuels' your body uses during dance

Dance will be fuelled by different compounds, derived from macronutrients, depending on the intensity, duration, training and nutritional intake of the dancer. These compounds can be metabolised to release energy either aerobically, where oxygen is needed or anaerobically, where energy can be produced without oxygen. This allows the body to fuel activity at different intensities economically; releasing as much energy from food eaten as possible. Your body has a series of systems which work in combination to optimise energy availability (EA) for the physical work being undertaken. As exercise duration increases, the contribution of each system gradually changes to ensure that our EA can be sustained as best as possible.

The stores of ATP in your body at any time are very small and only enough to sustain intense activity for a couple of seconds. Your body then has four options for energy to allow activity to be continued.

The four options for systems to fuel exercise have different time frames within which they operate. Starting with those fuelling very short highly intense dance activity and moving to those that sustain the less intense periods of longer duration energy can be supplied from:

1   Phosphocreatine (PCr): PCr is present in your cells and is broken down by an enzyme, creatine kinase, to phosphate and creatine. This phosphate can be added to adenosine diphosphate (ADP) to make ATP with the creation of an energy-rich bond. The energy can then be released when needed to carry out physical activity among other uses. The PCr stores in the cell will only result in energy release for a very short time – up to 10–15 seconds. After this, if activity continues, other energy supplies must be accessed. This system is anaerobic – it doesn't require the presence of oxygen. PCr will be resynthesised, once the high-intensity work is complete. It takes about 30 seconds to replace around 70% of the PCr. Levels are fully replaced after three to five minutes.

2   Glycogen. This is the carbohydrate store found in muscles and in the liver. It is used for high-intensity activity such as fast-paced jumping sections of classes and performances. Your glycogen stores are limited: they are estimated to be enough for less than two hours of high-intensity exercise (around 600 g in total between the liver and the muscles). Because glycogen has water stored with it, such that the 600 g has around 1800 g water associated with it, it results in a heavy energy store compared with fat, which is more energy dense (Fernández-Elias et al., 2015). The balance of energy stores in the body has evolved to allow dancers to be able to access fuels for different work intensities without adding large amounts of additional water weight to their bodies. Your body relies on you being able to eat carb-rich foods regularly to be able to replace your glycogen stores. Training allows you to spare your glycogen stores for use at the highest intensities by using fat as a fuel for higher-intensity

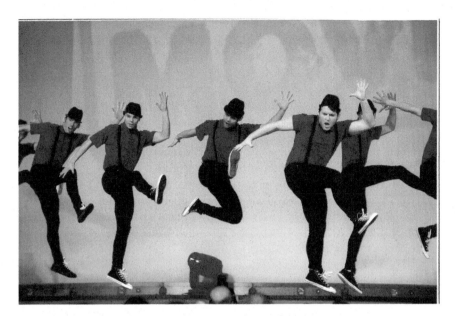

Photo 3.3 High-intensity dance is fuelled by carbohydrate.
Source: Photo courtesy of Jon Applegate

physical workloads than if you weren't trained, which is a very helpful adaptation (Holloszy & Coyle, 1984). Glycogen can be used both aerobically and anaerobically, so is not limited by the amount of oxygen you can deliver to your muscles.

3   Glucose. At all times you have glucose, a carb, in our circulation (blood). This can be used both aerobically and anaerobically. You can only use fuels anaerobically for up to three minutes. The energy for any dance activity over two to three minutes will need to be provided by aerobic metabolism, which limits the rate of energy production to how much oxygen you can deliver from your lungs to your muscles. Your blood glucose levels are constantly being depleted as energy is needed for the brain (which relies mainly on carbohydrate as its preferred fuel) and many body functions. Meals and snacks will replace these levels to keep your blood sugar levels in the normal healthy range. If necessary, you can convert glycogen back to glucose to make sure your blood glucose levels do not drop too low. In situations where there is a lack of carbohydrate, then protein can be broken down into carbohydrate.

4   Fats. Muscles contain fats (lipids), which are metabolised to release energy. Additionally, adipose tissue stores (body fat stores) are mainly in the form of triglycerides which can be broken down in the presence

of oxygen to release energy. This energy will supply the longer duration lower intensity parts of dance classes, rehearsals and performances as well as being part of the fuel that is used throughout the day and night.

Energy for movement and energy stores are both essential for survival. This is one potential reason why it is possible for the body to convert any spare carbohydrate into fat to be stored until needed, though it isn't the most efficient process and energy is needed for it. Any excess protein can also be converted into either carbohydrate or fat. The reverse is not the case: neither fat nor carbohydrate can be converted into protein.

Theoretically, fat can be converted into carbohydrate, but the amount that can potentially be converted is small and certainly isn't a process to rely on to maintain energy levels for high-intensity activity. Research consistently shows intense work can't be sustained when carb stores drop even when there are adequate fat stores available.

Practical point

It is very helpful to start re-fuelling with carbs as soon as possible after dance. See Chapter 4 for information on amounts and timings.

Those wishing to gain more detailed information on the area of fuel use at a cellular level will find the following text useful: Maughan, R.J., and Gleeson, M. (2010) *The Biochemical Basis of Sports Performance*. OUP Oxford.

V Introduction to the digestive system

It is useful to understand how digestion works to better plan the timing of what and when to take on board food to fuel dance and other activity.

The digestive system is the system in the body which processes food so it can be absorbed into the body. The nutrients released from food can be used for example for energy (macronutrients) and to support functions of the body (micronutrients).

What does the digestive system consist of?

The human digestive system consists of the gastrointestinal (GI) tract which begins with the mouth and progresses through the oesophagus (also spelt esophagus), stomach, small intestine (SI), large intestine (LI) also known as the colon, the very last parts of which are the rectum and anus. The liver, gall bladder and pancreas are also part of the digestive system, and different tissues are also involved. Tissues are group of cells that have similar structure and that work together as a unit. Examples in the digestive system are the layers which make up what is basically a tube with several layers which vary along the length of the tube but including muscle, connective tissue and secretory cells and expand at the stomach, which is a sac which can typically hold around 800 ml. The SI is around 6 m in length with a diameter of about 2.4 cm. The LI is around 1.5 m long and has a diameter of 3–8 cm. This length is necessary to allow digestion to take place effectively. The role of the digestive system is, the name implies, to digest and absorb nutrients. This process also requires input from the salivary glands, the liver and pancreas, and in most people also the gall bladder (which stores bile, produced by the liver, which helps in the digestion of fat) (Figures 3.3 and 3.4).

What happens in digestion and why does it matter for dancers?

It is useful to consider how different parts of the digestive system contribute to the process of digestion, as this can potentially help with getting timing

MOUTH, PHARYNX AND ESOPHAGUS

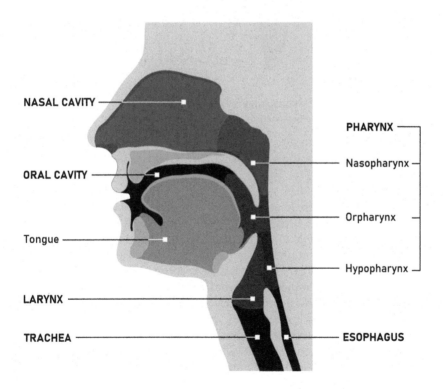

Figure 3.3 The digestive system from the mouth to the oesophagus.
Credit: logika600/Shutterstock.com

Digestive system

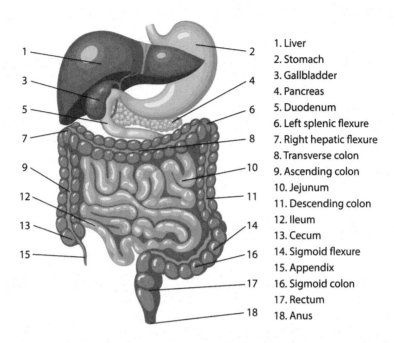

1. Liver
2. Stomach
3. Gallbladder
4. Pancreas
5. Duodenum
6. Left splenic flexure
7. Right hepatic flexure
8. Transverse colon
9. Ascending colon
10. Jejunum
11. Descending colon
12. Ileum
13. Cecum
14. Sigmoid flexure
15. Appendix
16. Sigmoid colon
17. Rectum
18. Anus

Figure 3.4 The digestive system from the stomach onwards.
Credit: Olga Bolbot/Shutterstock.com

of meals and snacks best for performance, and also specific points for the dancer.

- *The mouth* is where digestion begins, specifically digestion of carbo-hydrates. Chewing breaks the food into very small particles which are then more accessible to the enzymes further down the GI tract. Amyl-ase, an enzyme contained in saliva, breaks down starch, a complex car-bohydrate, into sugars which can be absorbed into the body and used for energy. Even though only a small proportion, around 5%, of the car-bohydrate in food or drink is digested in the mouth, this can still impact on energy and performance, for example carbohydrate mouth rinses have been shown to improve sports performance (Stellingwerff & Cox, 2014). Saliva also contains lipase which breaks down small amounts of some types of fats and trace amounts of proteases to contribute to pro-tein break down.
- *The mouth and stomach* also have a role in assessing what is being ingested and contributing to the sense of fullness, both satiation,

which is the sense of being full that results in a meal ending, and satiety, which is the feeling of fullness/lack of hunger which contributes to when we next feel the need to eat. The volume of food, the texture and amount of chewing needed, the amount of fluid in/with the food, the amount of fibre and the nutrient density all contribute to this. Dancers who often have a packed schedule are not always able to act on these cues, and there is value in finding ways to eat enough in the times available to supply the body with the nutrients it needs.

- *In the stomach*, the release of acid and enzymes continues the digestion process started in the mouth, with the focus particularly on getting protein digestion underway. The partially digested food, known as chyme, starts to leave the stomach after a minimum of 40 minutes and moves into the SI where digestion continues, and most of the nutrient absorption takes place. Dancers typically have to dance while digestion is underway but are likely to find energy levels better if at least an hour can elapse between eating and dance so the stomach has at least partially emptied. There is a need for increased blood flow to the gut for digestion and to muscles for activity. Practice allows the body to adapt, but it is still advisable, if possible, to have a break between eating and dancing.
- The first part of the SI is called the *duodenum* and is about 20–25 cm long. The chyme is now mixed with digestive enzymes produced by the pancreas, which is located very close by, and transported via ducts into the SI. The digestive enzymes produced by the pancreas include proteases which break down proteins for absorption and amylases and lipases which undertake the digestion of carbohydrates and fats respectively. As fat is not water soluble, it is harder to digest than carbohydrates and proteins.
- Bile is also released into the duodenum. Bile, produced by the liver, contains bile acids which enhance fat digestion, as well as bile salts which contribute to the absorption of fat-soluble vitamins. Overall bile is alkaline and helps to neutralise the chyme, which is acidic. The duodenum also contains Brunner's glands which produce a mucus-rich alkaline secretion. This secretion has an important role in neutralising chyme together with bicarbonate from the pancreas. A small amount of nutrient absorption occurs in the duodenum, but the majority occurs in the second part of the SI.
- The second part of the SI is the *jejunum*. It is about 2.5 m long, and, as with the entire SI, the surface is made up of many tiny folds in finger-like villi that massively increase its surface area. In the jejunum, the breakdown products of carbohydrates, proteins and fats are absorbed across the villi and into the blood stream for transportation to the cells of the body. And, of course, the GI tract itself also needs a good supply of nutrients to stay healthy.

- The final part of the SI is the *ileum*, around 3.5 m long. This is where the final parts of digestive absorption take place. The ileum re-absorbs bile acids, as well as absorbing some fluid, and vitamin B-12.
- The role of the LI which is approximately 1.5 m long is to absorb water and electrolytes – minerals such as sodium and potassium as well as allow the processing of the residue of food left after digestion in the SI. In the LI are the billions of bacteria with an overall composition unique to each of us that can metabolise many types of fibre either partially or totally with the production of fatty acids which are then available to us. Inadequate fluid – see the chapter on hydration – can increase the risk of constipation, which is unhelpful for feeling energised.
- The microbiome is the term used for the population of bacteria we have in the LI. Research over the last few years has shown many ways in which the composition of the population can impact on our health and even influence our energy levels (Mach & Fuster-Botella, 2017).
- As well as producing bile the liver also has a role in vitamin D metabolism which impacts on energy (Roy et al., 2014) and muscle fatigue (de Rezende Araújo II et al., 2020).
- The pancreas produces digestive enzymes – this is known as the exocrine system. It also has an endocrine role – the systems which involve hormones within the body. The endocrine role of the pancreas is to produce insulin which is crucial to regulating your blood glucose (sugar) levels. When there is insufficient insulin, or the insulin produced doesn't work effectively the result is diabetes mellitus. Where insulin production stops almost completely, the result is Type 1 diabetes, which usually starts before the age of 30. There have been a number of high-performing athletes and dancers with Type 1 diabetes – more on this is covered in Chapter 13. Cystic fibrosis can also result in Type 1 diabetes. Unfortunately, extreme intakes of alcohol or drugs can also damage the pancreas and result in problems with insulin production.

How long does digestion take?

While a meal made up only of carbohydrates – sugars and starches – can be digested and absorbed upwards of two hours from the time it is eaten, meals rich in protein will take longer, with high-fat meals taking longest, up to six hours or so. Anxiety usually delays the process of digestion and dancers are advised to bear this in mind when facing challenging situations such as auditions, assessments and performances, and allow longer than normal between eating and dancing.

Research in sport has focussed on how much carbohydrate and protein can be absorbed in specific amounts of time to support those undertaking endurance activities to perform at their best. This information can be useful to dancers as consuming higher amounts may result in problems with the digestive system. Food eaten close to physical activity is best if it is low in fat to minimise the time taken to digest it. For this reason, recommendations on maximum amounts of macronutrients focus on carbs and proteins and not fats.

Are there any limits to how much carbohydrate the dancer can tolerate?

The maximum amount of one type of carb that can be absorbed per hour is around 60 g. An amount of 30–60 g/hour is recommended for those undertaking endurance exercise of 1–2.5 hours duration including 'stop start' type activity (Jeukendrup 2014). Dancers are typically not used to taking nutrition on board during performances, although intervals and time off stage do provide opportunities in theory. There is certainly currently no culture of planning any level of nutrient intake during classes, though this is an option to look at for the future. With practicalities such as safety in studios as a major consideration, this is not a straightforward discussion. It is possible to absorb more than 60 g carbohydrate per hour if a combination of different types is used. From mixed sources, for example a combination of glucose and fructose then it can be possible for the body to absorb up to 90 g carb per hour. Dancers are unlikely to need this amount under most circumstances, though for some individuals in specific situations, it could be relevant, for example technical and dress rehearsals for productions with a substantial amount of high-intensity dance for some individuals due to the dances they are in. This area will be looked at in more detail in Chapter 4.

Is there a maximum amount of protein to take in one meal/snack?

There is evidence that around 20 g protein is the best amount in one go after exercise if muscle fibre synthesis is the aim (Witard et al., 2014). Otherwise spreading protein across meals and snacks in the day, with 20–30 g at main meals, is a practical way of achieving your protein goals. This will be looked at in detail in Chapter 5.

Although there are guidelines as to maximum amounts of macronutrients to include at meals, there can be benefits to considering your own needs and how these vary from day to day. This is explored in the next sections.

VI The FITT self-test

The FITT principles were originally used for those planning training programmes for themselves to make sure they had thought through all the relevant factors. The FITT principles can also be useful to dancers when considering their energy and nutrient needs for the day and week. Although schedules can, and do, change, spending some time planning is helpful to allow you to meet your requirements. In particular, your carb needs vary depending on the amount, duration and intensity of activity, so thinking about each of the principles below can be helpful before moving into Chapter 4 and focussing on carbs. Protein needs also vary slightly according to your current goals – this will be looked at in Chapter 5.

Frequency: Do you have classes/rehearsals/performances/additional training daily (with a rest day), or is it less frequent, perhaps two to four times per week?

Intensity: How hard is your body working? Does the activity increase heart rate and cause rapid breathing? Examples: jumping sequences in ballet, fast tap routines, contemporary pieces involving covering distance fast. Does the activity require sustained muscular strength without much movement? This would include ballet barre work, slow centre work and partner work.

Timing: How much time (minutes/hours) do you spend dancing or supplemental activity per day? Although it is still tiring to be learning new choreography, actual time dancing is the important factor for considering energy needs, so try and separate actual dance from standing time.

Type of activity: Different styles of dance and supplemental training have different energy and nutrient needs: if you are working at building strength pay particular attention to protein requirements – see Chapter 5.

VII Working out your energy requirements

This is a somewhat theoretical, numerical section, and readers who have struggled with their relationship with food may prefer to focus more on practical sections and move ahead to section VI of this chapter. The information included here is to provide a reference source, as there are so many myths and half-truths surrounding the subject of nutrition.

It is useful to start with some brief definitions around metabolism and metabolic rate:

Metabolism is the chemical processes during which your body converts nutrients from food and drinks into energy, converts food into the structural compounds needed for health, and eliminates waste products from the body. Your basal metabolic rate (BMR): this is the amount of energy required for the body at complete rest, lying down, in the fasted state (as digesting food also requires energy, and produces heat). It is impacted mainly by age and body composition. There is also a genetic element too, though more data are needed to clarify this.

You may see reference to resting metabolic rate (RMR). This would be measured lying completely still and relaxed but doesn't require you to be fasted, so it will include the energy you are using to digest food.

Total energy expenditure (TEE): the amount of energy an individual uses in 24 hours. This includes the BMR, plus the energy used in digestion, plus that for all movement undertaken (Westerterp, 2013). While it is possible to estimate your energy requirements, log your intake and measure your energy expenditure with varying degrees of accuracy, you are advised to think carefully about whether, and how it would be useful for you. Nutrition is so much more than calories/kilojoules in and out, and focussing on calories can make it hard to keep in mind the importance of the whole range of both macro- and micronutrients you need to perform at your best.

Research measuring actual energy expenditure, from heat production, in a specialised chamber, called a calorimeter, has allowed scientists to produce equations to predict BMR without having to actually measure it. The different equations given below all allow you to estimate your BMR. They were derived in different populations so are all slightly different.

There are several different predictive equations for BMR, the one derived by Harris and Benedict known as the Harris-Benedict equation is:

Males: kcal per day = 66.4730 + 13.7516W + 5.0033S − 6.7750A
Females: kcal per day = 665.0955 + 9.5634W + 1.8496S − 4.6756A
W-weight (kg), H-Height (cm), A-Age (years)
Be very careful to use the correct units, especially for height – cm not metres.

The equations created by Schofield in 1985 and finally by Henry (Henry, 2005) are given here:

Gender Equation Descriptive equation for BMR (MJ/24 h) ages 18–30
Male Schofield BMR = 0.063 × (Weight) + 2.896
Henry BMR = 0.0669 × (Weight) + 2.28
Female Schofield BMR = 0.062 × (Weight) + 2.036
Henry BMR = 0.0546 x (Weight) +2.33

The Cunningham equation requires having an estimate of your lean body mass, rather than your total weight, as the equation is: BMR (kcal/day) = 500 + 22 (LBM) (Cunningham, 1980). As we will see in Chapter 9, there are limitations to measuring body composition, but it is possible to get an estimate from skinfold thickness measurements or BIA (Bioelectrical impedance analysis) if the methods are followed carefully.

Research in athletes has suggested that the Harris-Benedict equation is the most useful for male athletes, and less useful for females, while the Cunningham equation has been suggested to be the most useful for female athletes (Jagim et al., 2018).

The Owen equation for non-athletes is: RMR = 795 + (7.18 × weight kg).

For athletes is: RMR = 50.4 + (21.1 × weight kg). It has been shown to be useful for Hispanic women (Miller et al., 2013) and in some disabilities, see Chapter 9. These RMR values are kcal/day.

There are further equations which can be useful such as the Mifflin St Jeor equations for REE (kcal/day) rather than BMR: REE (males) = 10 × weight (kg) + 6.25 × height (cm) −5 × age (y) + 5; REE (females) = 10 × weight (kg) + 6.25 × height (cm) − 5 × age (y) − 161 (Mifflin et al., 1990).

Once you have an estimate for your BMR, you can then multiply this by a physical activity level (PAL) factor to predict likely total energy requirements for a day. Its best to be careful when working through BMR calculations as any error will be multiplied when you look at estimates for a day's energy needs.

The FAO has categorised PAL as follows:
The minimum for extremely sedentary individuals: BMR × 1.2
Days that are sedentary - lightly activity: BMR × 1.4-1.69
Days that are active or moderately active: BMR × 1.7-1.99
Days that are vigorous or vigorously active: BMR × 2-2.4
Dancers are likely to spend most dance days at a PAL of at least 1.75, and at around 2.0 on many days.
The highest PAL values have been shown in endurance events, for example in 3 weeks of competitive cycling, and in dragging sleds across the Arctic PAL values of 4.5–4.7 were seen.

(United Nations/FAO 2001)

There has been considerable research into the minimum amounts of energy that are enough for athletes. This is expressed as EA per kg fat-free mass (FFM), so this needs to be the first step if there is concern over intake. A minimum of 45 kcal/kg FFM is recommended for athletes – and dancers (Burke et al., 2018). This will be discussed in more detail in Chapter 11.

A quick note on trackers such as heart rate monitors. Whether worn on the chest or as a watch these take heart rate data and using predictive equations to estimate TEE. While the heart rate tracking is reported as being accurate, so far the data on energy expenditure lack accuracy (Fuller et al., 2020).

VIII Energy needs for classes and rehearsals

Energy needs are considered in this section and the next, again to see what the evidence is for energy requirements for different styles of dance. This is not to suggest any dancer should be calorie counting; data are here to confirm that all dance is energy demanding, and meeting your energy needs allows you to perform at your best.

Energy needs vary between activities and from day to day

Your energy needs for dance are not constant. A pre-professional student may be taking up to six or seven classes daily, while professionals will be taking class and will then be in rehearsals and/or performances. For those in training even if all your classes are the same genre, which is rare as most dance training covers multiple genres, there will be variation in the energy requirements from class to class. Dance in general is recognised to be an 'intermittent sprint' activity. In other words, there are sections of any class/ rehearsal/performance that are slower, less intense, and those which are fast and intense, and of course a spectrum between these extremes. The lower-intensity sections are recognised as aerobic – where fats and carbohydrates are metabolised when oxygen is present as we saw earlier. Fats require more oxygen to release energy than carbohydrates do, but reserves are greater. As dance intensity increases and energy requirements increase, it becomes impossible for enough oxygen to reach the muscles to allow fats or carbohy-drates to be metabolised aerobically. Anaerobic metabolism now becomes more important, where carbohydrates can be metabolised without oxygen to supply energy for dance. As discussed earlier, anaerobic metabolism of carbohydrate can be used to fuel high-intensity dance for up to about two minutes. The body is unable to sustain anaerobic metabolism beyond this point and intensity will need to be reduced back into the aerobic zone.

Research data on energy use in dance

Dance of all genres demonstrates the use of short periods of high-intensity dance and longer periods of moderate- or low-intensity dance, but the time spent in each has been demonstrated to vary, at least when comparing ballet and contemporary dance. Ballet had longer periods of high- to very high-intensity exercise and longer periods at rest compared with more continu-ous moderate-intensity activity in contemporary dance (Wyon et al., 2011). Shaw et al., (2021) conclude that more clarity in data collection and more research is needed even when looking only at professional ballet dancers.

From the limited research which has focussed mainly on ballet and con-temporary, dance energy requirements of classes can be very different to rehearsals, the latter being more energy demanding, in particular dress re-hearsals. There is a further step up to performances. The demands of classes also vary from year to year in pre-professional training (Beck et al., 2018). As might be expected training days have been shown to be more energy demanding than weekend days in pre-professional ballet students. On week-days, the average energy output of this group (average age 19 years) was 2,400 kcal/day; at weekends, it was 2,110 kcal/day (Civil et al., 2019).

A similar study in female pre-professional contemporary dance students reported weekday energy expenditure to be an average of 2,720 kcal/ day on weekdays and 2,630 kcal/day at weekends (Brown et al., 2017)

Research on tap dance in 1979 looked at a small group of female beginners and intermediates doing two routines and concluded the energy required was similar to that for ballroom dance such as waltz, foxtrot and rumba (Noble & Howley, 1979). Recent research has noted tap to be much more demanding than contem-porary dance or ballet, with heart rates up to 84% of maximum, and around 350 kcal/hour being used in the session which simulated a tap class (Oliveira et al., 2010). Ballroom dance has been shown to use an average of 360 kcal/hour for recreational dancers, waltz and foxtrot being lower than swing (320 and 480 kcal/ hour) (Lankford et al., 2014). A study of Japanese professional ballroom dancers showed heart rates to be in the range defined as 'highly physically demanding' at over 150 beats/minute (Hirose et al., 2021). Male ballroom dancers have been estimated to use over 12 kcal/minute, which equates to over 700 kcal/hour if continuous, with females estimated to use over 8 kcal/minute (around 500 kcal/hour) (Blanksby & Reidy, 1988; Massidda et al., 2011): these are extremely high requirements and further data are needed on sustained use. Musical theatre energy use lacks data, but physiological demands have been shown to be high for both dancing alone and singing and dancing combined, and musical theatre performers to have greater aerobic fitness than other dance theatre genres (Stephens & Wyon, 2020). Pilates energy use depends on the type of class, with female energy use estimated at around 115 kcal/hour for a mat class, and 155 kcal/hour using Reformer equipment (de Souza Andrade et al., 2021). From these data you can see that although there is variation, dance requires considerable amounts of energy per hour. It is important to also note that when you stop any activity, your metabolism doesn't immediately return back to resting levels.

A summary of estimated requirements for different styles of dance is shown in Table 3.2

Table 3.2 Estimated approximate energy requirements for dance: these will vary according to age, weight, fitness and experience

Style of dance	Energy (kcal) needed per hour continuous dance: average	Energy (kcal) needed per hour continuous dance males	Energy (kcal) needed per hour continuous dance females
Ballet: low intensity		350	240
Ballet: moderate intensity		360	280
Ballet: high intensity		500	350
Contemporary – medium intensity/*warm up*	300 *Students: 220* *Professionals: 265*		
Contemporary centre work	Students: 340 Professionals: 380		
Tap	350		
Ballroom: recreational dancers, waltz, foxtrot	320		
Ballroom: recreational dancers, swing dance	480		
Dance sport Latin		251	160
Pilates			Reformer: 155 Mat: 116
Simulated Latin American dance		8–14 kcal/minute	6–8 kcal/minute
Folk		840	600

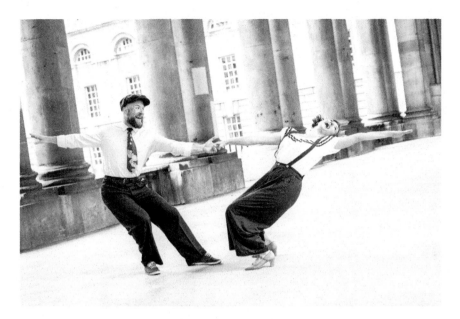

Photo 3.4 Dance is characterised by movement at varying intensities.
Source: Photo courtesy of Helen Rimell

For comparison, a report by Vaz et al (2005) provides data on estimated energy requirements for non-dance activities.
Because calories are the energy in macronutrients but take no account of other nutrients, tracking calories is of very limited use for dancers and gives almost no indication of how well food intake meets requirements. Rather than focussing on numerical energy needs – calories – dancers are advised to think about the amounts of foods rich in protein, carbs and fats that will meet their needs and follow this up in the next three chapters.

Timing of meals/snacks

While liquids begin to leave the stomach within a few minutes of drinking, food only begins to leave the stomach after at least 40 minutes. Fibre, protein and particularly fat will slow down the speed food leaves the stomach, and a large high fat meal can take six hours, although typically a meal will take two to four hours to leave the stomach completely. There is then a further one to two hours or more needed for digestion and absorption of nutrients in the SI. Dancers generally can train, rehearse and perform while digestion is ongoing, however as blood flow is diverted to the gut for 1.5–2 hours after eating a meal, with the peak at 20–40 minutes after a meal allowing at least 40 minutes between eating and dancing is likely to

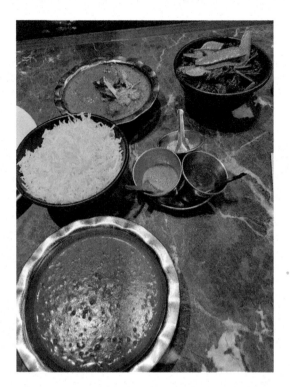

Photo 3.5 Photo Jasmine Challis.

minimise any impacts of this. Dancing while hungry is not recommended, so the aim is to have a break of at least 40 minutes between food and dance (or other physical activity) but then to be able to have a snack within two to three hours, and a meal within four to six hours, though this gap can be a little longer if one to two nutritious snacks can be fitted in to the schedule.

The fact that liquids can be absorbed more quickly than solids means that timing and choice of drinks can be an important part of your nutrition strategy. Chapter 7 looks at hydration, but liquids can also contribute to nutritional intake. Using milk or an alternative with a reasonable protein content – look for at least 2 g/100 ml – or yoghurt as the basis for a smoothie can supply valuable nutrition that can be digested more quickly than solid food and help you meet your nutrition needs. See the recipes section for ideas on smoothie recipes.

Dancers usually cope well with fitting nutritious snacks into small breaks in their dance schedule. Meals take a little more planning, and it may work best to split them into two if dance goes across your normal meal times. Always having an extra snack or two in your bag means that even if schedules change at very short notice you are able to re-fuel and maintain energy levels as best as possible.

IX Energy needs and timing for performance days

Most research is laboratory based, requiring dancers to carry out pre-planned routines to be able to repeat measurements. Data derived from this are of course useful, but performance data, when available, will help practical understanding of dancers' needs. One study published in 2019 looking at female Korean ballet dancers before and after performance days estimated their average TEE to be over 3,000 kcal/day (Kim et al., 2019). A review by Beck in 2015 highlights the fact that there is an increase in energy demands from training/rehearsals to performances (Beck et al., 2015). Nutrition alone can't increase your strength and stamina to cope with performances, but meeting your energy needs from food will help you to maintain your performance energy levels. The many severe consequences of under nutrition include increased risk of injury. This is explored in Chapter 11.

When to eat on performance days

Performance day schedules can make it difficult to eat at your normal times, and the time you have for eating may be less than usual, especially if there are two or even three performances in one day. Starting with a good breakfast, and including some protein – porridge made with milk and with added nuts/ seeds and fruit is a good option; another option tried and tested by many dancers is scrambled eggs or tofu and toast, with avocado and some veggies, e.g. tomatoes/spinach. Both will set you up for the day ahead by providing a good range of nutrients. However, it is never good to experiment on performance days, so always try out different options before performance days.

To allow time for digestion dancers are advised to eat at least 1.5–2 hours before performances to ensure good energy levels for the performance. Eating a meal three to four hours before a performance is optimal for many, though those with a faster digestion may be able to eat meals with less of a gap. Lighter meals are usually tolerated 1.5–2 hours before a performance and snacks up to about an hour before a performance. If you have a matinee performance, then a good breakfast followed by an early lunch is a great strategy. Eat a snack as soon as you can after the performance to re-fuel, or, if you have an evening performance, then a meal in the break between performances is your best option: aim for different foods to those you had at lunch but nothing high fat as this will be slow to digest. Pastry and fried food, including chips, are not ideal, and pizza is likely to be slow to digest too; if options are limited, then a chicken or vegetarian burger (easy on the mayo) are better options than a pie and chips. If you are on tour, then researching your options and ordering ahead will give the best chance to meet your needs. If you are very anxious, then digestion may be slower than

Table 3.3 Sample schedule for meals and snacks for a day with one or two performances

	Matinee and evening	Evening only
Breakfast examples	Overnight oats or porridge with milk/yoghurt, nuts/ seeds, fruit/dried fruit OR Eggs/tofu with avo/spread and toast with veggies	Overnight oats or porridge with milk/yoghurt, nuts/ seeds, fruit/dried fruit OR Eggs/tofu with avo/spread and toast with veggies
Snack if needed, examples	Fruit/bar/nuts/milky coffee	Fruit/bar/nuts/milky coffee
Lunch examples	Wrap/sandwich with fruit/yoghurt	Hot meal – all food groups
Mid-late afternoon	Snack straight after matinee if no evening performance otherwise early meal	Light meal 1.5–2 hours before performance
Evening/late evening	Dinner at normal time/ snack meal after evening performance	Snack/meal after performance depending on your needs

normal, so allow a bigger gap between eating and performance. Your goal is to arrive on stage neither full nor hungry, and with great energy levels. A suggested schedule for performance days is shown in Table 3.3.

X Energy needs for rest days and injuries and holidays

Rest days

First, it's essential to take rest days. The aim is to take at least one rest day per week. This allows your body time to recover from training, rehearsals and performances. Rest days offer a chance to continue the re-fuelling process, and to make sure you are well-fuelled for the next day of dance. While you may not need as much energy from macronutrients on rest days as dance days, what is certain is that you won't benefit from restricting your intake either. If you can rely on appetite, then that is great for meeting your needs. If your schedule or experiences make it challenging to rely on appetite then using the guidance in the chapters on individual macronutrients is another option. What is helpful is to continue to focus on varied, nutrient-rich foods, especially if you have struggled to meet your needs over the previous few days. If your rest day(s) are at weekends, then it can be helpful to think of Saturday as a day to re-fuel from the week that has gone and Sunday as a day to ensure glycogen stores are kept topped up ready for work to begin on Monday. If you have only one rest day, whenever that is, then focussing on meeting protein needs, as these will not drop dramatically on a rest day, together with appropriate carbs and fats, with the majority of your intake spread evenly over three meals, together with a smaller amount in at least one snack, is going to help the 're-fuelling and pre-fuelling' processes.

Injuries

Although activity may be reduced if you have an injury, your energy intake needs to be adequate to allow healing to take place. This will be above your requirements at rest, but the exact amount will depend on the injury, treatment and what activity you are able to do and is likely to vary from day to day. Additionally, protein will be needed for many injuries to heal, along with other nutrients depending on the site of the injury. If you are struggling psychologically after injury, this may impact on appetite and result in either reduced intake, especially if you are in pain, or alternatively may result in comfort/emotional eating. Seek support if you are struggling, and aim to focus on fuel to allow optimal healing in your recovery process. Many dancers will be anxious about changes in body composition if activity is reduced significantly. Any changes will be minimised by focussing on the nutrients you need and maintaining attention on what you can control. This area is looked at in more detail in Chapter 11.

Holidays and other changes to routine

Food on holidays is typically different to day-to-day food, whether you have travelled abroad, locally, or are taking time off at home. Opportunities to enjoy different foods can be a time to broaden your range of foods or recipes. This is likely to be beneficial by making food more interesting and also possibly improving nutrient intake, depending on your normal day-to-day food choices.

Be mindful that if your schedule changes dramatically for more than a day or so, and meal times change, it can be harder to respond to appetite, and this can impact on energy levels as well as possibly on body composition, which may make resuming normal training and performances harder. This is not a given but means that a little planning can be useful to avoid unintended outcomes. One additional factor that may change is that alcohol intakes can increase on holiday – think about how best to manage this for your upcoming schedule for health, well-being and performance once the holiday is over.

Many dancers continue exercise in some form over their holidays. Whatever your plans are, meeting your energy needs should be included. Shifting the balance of macronutrients slightly more towards fats temporarily, and including more high-sugar products rather than less-refined choices, is unlikely to cause problems in the longer term when normal dance activity resumes, though there is a lack of data on this. Not surprisingly the body is able to adapt to changes in macronutrient provision but does need a few days from what is known currently.

There are many events in performers' lives that can impact on energy requirements. Your body is able to tolerate small differences where intake and output are not exactly matched and still maintain good energy levels, providing fluctuations allow good glycogen repletion and overall, on average, energy requirements are met. You are still advised to meet requirements as consistently as possible – fuelling your workload. The next three chapters look in detail at each macronutrient and cover both theory and practical advice on meeting your requirements for each macronutrient.

XI Resources

Bytomski, J.R. (2018) Fueling for performance, *Sports Health*, 10(1), pp.47–53. https://www.nature.com/scitable/topicpage/nutrient-utilization-in-humans-metabolism-pathways-14234029/.
Maughan, R.J., and Gleeson, M. (2010) *The Biochemical Basis of Sports Performance*. OUP Oxford.

XII Learning outcomes

After reading this chapter, the reader should be able to:

1   Identify the macronutrients important for dancers, and their use.
2   Explain the different systems for replenish ATP stores and when each is used.
3   Discuss the suitability of different meals and snacks before training and performance.

References

Beck, S., Redding, E. and Wyon, M.A. (2015) Methodological considerations for documenting the energy demand of dance activity: A review, *Frontiers in Psychology*, 6, pp.568.
Beck, S., Wyon, M.A. and Redding, E. (2018) Changes in energy demand of dance activity and cardiorespiratory fitness during 1 year of vocational contemporary dance training, *The Journal of Strength & Conditioning Research,* 32(3), pp.841–848.
Blanksby, B.A. and Reidy, P.W. (1988) Heart rate and estimated energy expenditure during ballroom dancing, *British Journal of Sports Medicine*, 22(2), pp.57–60.
Brown, M.A. et al. (2017) Energy intake and energy expenditure of pre-professional female contemporary dancers, *PLoS One*, 12(2), pp.e0171998.
Burke, L.M. et al. (2018) Pitfalls of conducting and interpreting estimates of energy availability in free-living athletes, *International Journal of Sport Nutrition and Exercise Metabolism*, 28(4), pp.350–363.
Bytomski, J.R. (2018) Fueling for performance, *Sports Health*, 10(1), pp.47–53.
Civil, R. et al. (2019) Assessment of dietary intake, energy status, and factors associated with RED-S in vocational female ballet students, *Frontiers in Nutrition*, 5, p.136.

Cunningham, J.J. (1980) A reanalysis of the factors influencing basal metabolic rate in normal adults, *The American Journal of Clinical Nutrition*, 33(11), pp.2372–2374.

de Rezende Araújo, Iris Iasmine et al. (2020) The relationship between vitamin D levels, injury and muscle function in adolescent dancers, *International Journal of Sports Medicine*, 41(06), pp.360–364.

Fernández-Elías, V.E. et al. (2015) Relationship between muscle water and glycogen recovery after prolonged exercise in the heat in humans, *European Journal of Applied Physiology,* 115(9), pp.1919–1926.

Fuller, D. et al. (2020) Reliability and validity of commercially available wearable devices for measuring steps, energy expenditure, and heart rate: Systematic review, *JMIR mHealth and uHealth*, 8(9), pp.e18694.

Henry, C. (2005) Basal metabolic rate studies in humans: Measurement and development of new equations, *Public Health Nutrition*, 8(7a), pp.1133–1152.

Hirose, T. et al. (2021) Heart rate in ballroom dance in Japanese professional dancers, *Statistics*, 60, pp.90sec.

Holloszy, J.O. and Coyle, E.F. (1984) Adaptations of skeletal muscle to endurance exercise and their metabolic consequences, *Journal of Applied Physiology*, 56(4), pp.831–838.

Jagim, A.R. et al. (2018) Accuracy of resting metabolic rate prediction equations in athletes, *The Journal of Strength & Conditioning Research*, 32(7), pp.1875–1881.

Jeukendrup, A. (2014) A step towards personalized sports nutrition: Carbohydrate intake during exercise, *Sports Medicine*, 44(1), pp.25–33.

Kim, S.Y. et al. (2019) Changes in body composition, energy metabolism, and appetite-regulating hormones in Korean professional female ballet dancers before and after ballet performance, *Journal of Dance Medicine & Science,* 23(4), pp.173–180.

Lanham-New, S. et al. (2019) *Introduction to human nutrition 3rd edition*, The Nutrition Society Textbook Series. Wiley Blackwell, Chichester, UK.

Lankford, D.E. et al. (2014) The energy expenditure of recreational ballroom dance, *International Journal of Exercise Science*, 7(3), pp.228.

Mach, N. and Fuster-Botella, D. (2017) Endurance exercise and gut microbiota: A review, *Journal of Sport and Health Science*, 6(2), pp.179–197.

Massidda, M. et al. (2011) Energy expenditure during competitive Latin American dancing simulation, *Medical Problems of Performing Artists*, 26(4), pp.206–210.

Mifflin, M.D. et al. (1990) A new predictive equation for resting energy expenditure in healthy individuals, *The American Journal of Clinical Nutrition*, 51(2), pp.241–247.

Miller, S., Milliron, B. and Woolf, K. (2013) Common prediction equations overestimate measured resting metabolic rate in young Hispanic women, *Topics in Clinical Nutrition*, 28(2), pp.120.

Noble, R.M. and Howley, E.T. (1979) The energy requirement of selected tap dance routines, Research Quarterly, *American Alliance for Health, Physical Education, Recreation and Dance*, 50(3), pp.438–442.

Oliveira, S.M. et al. (2010) Physiological responses to a tap dance choreography: Comparisons with graded exercise test and prescription recommendations, *The Journal of Strength & Conditioning Research,* 24(7), pp.1954–1959.

Oosthuyse, T., Carstens, M. and Millen, A.M. (2015) Ingesting isomaltulose versus fructose-maltodextrin during prolonged moderate-heavy exercise increases fat oxidation but impairs gastrointestinal comfort and cycling performance,

International Journal of Sport Nutrition and Exercise Metabolism, 25(5), pp.427–438.

Pasiakos, S.M. et al. (2014) Whole-body protein turnover response to short-term high-protein diets during weight loss: A randomized controlled trial, *International Journal of Obesity*, 38(7), pp.1015–1018.

Romijn, J.A. et al. (1993) Regulation of endogenous fat and carbohydrate metabolism in relation to exercise intensity and duration, *American Journal of Physiology-Endocrinology and Metabolism*, 265(3), pp.E380–E391.

Roy, S. et al. (2014) Correction of low vitamin D improves fatigue: Effect of correction of low vitamin D in fatigue study (EViDiF study), *North American Journal of Medical Sciences*, 6(8), p.396.

Shaw, J.W. et al. (2021) The activity demands and physiological responses observed in professional ballet: A systematic review, *The Journal of Sport and Exercise Science*, 5(4), pp.254–269.

Stellingwerff, T. and Cox, G.R. (2014) Systematic review: Carbohydrate supplementation on exercise performance or capacity of varying durations, *Applied Physiology, Nutrition, and Metabolism*, 39(9), pp.998–1011.

Stephens, N. and Wyon, M. (2020) Physiological characteristics of musical theatre performers and the effect on cardiorespiratory demand whilst singing and dancing, *Medical Problems of Performing Artists*, 35(1), pp.54–58.

Thomas, D.T., Erdman, K.A. and Burke, L.M. (2016) Position of the academy of nutrition and dietetics, dietitians of Canada, and the American College of Sports Medicine: Nutrition and athletic performance, *Journal of the Academy of Nutrition and Dietetics*, 116(3), pp.501–528.

United Nations University and World Health Organization (2004) Human Energy Requirements: Report of a Joint FAO/WHO/UNU Expert Consultation: Rome, 17–24 October 2001, *Food & Agriculture Org*, Technical Report Series No. 1, pp.35–50.

Vaz, M. et al. (2005) A compilation of energy costs of physical activities, *Public Health Nutrition*, 8(7a), pp.1153–1183.

Westerterp, K.R. (2013) Physical activity and physical activity induced energy expenditure in humans: Measurement, determinants, and effects, *Frontiers in Physiology*, 4, p.90.

Witard, O.C. et al. (2014) Myofibrillar muscle protein synthesis rates subsequent to a meal in response to increasing doses of whey protein at rest and after resistance exercise, *The American Journal of Clinical Nutrition*, 99(1), pp.86–95.

Wyon, M.A. et al. (2011) Time motion and video analysis of classical ballet and contemporary dance performance, *International Journal of Sports Medicine*, 32(11), pp.851–855.

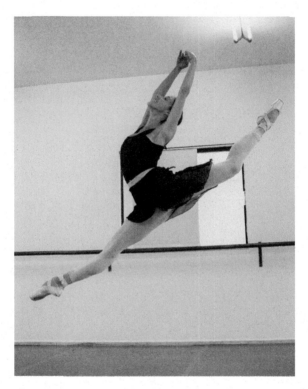

Photo 4.1 Photo courtesy of Arthur Giglioli.

4 Carbohydrate for training and performance

Contents

Carbohydrate myth	Carbohydrate reality
You shouldn't eat carbohydrate-rich foods in the evening	Glycogen (muscle energy) stores are depleted after dance, refuelling in the evening replenish stores to support dance the next day.
You can get all the carbs you need from vegetables and fruit	Most vegetables contain only small amounts of carb. Although fruit is a good source of carbs, the effect on gut and teeth of taking a very high fruit diet (over five portions per day) makes this inadvisable.
Bread is the same as sugar	Bread, especially wholegrain varieties, contributes to protein intake and is a source of B vitamins, iron and other minerals as well as carbohydrates and is digested more slowly than sugar.

DOI: 10.4324/9781003219002-4

I Introduction: carbohydrate utilisation during dance

Your brain needs carbohydrate to help you decipher that tricky step, while your muscles need carbohydrate to master it. As discussed in Chapter 3, carbohydrates are one of the two macronutrients the body relies on to metabolise for energy, the other being lipids (fats). Of these two, carbohydrate is the main energy-providing nutrient for dancers. Protein can, in theory, be used for energy; however, for reasons that are discussed in Chapter 5, this is not your best option.

Together, glucose and its stored form glycogen provide about half of the energy used by your brain, muscles and body tissues over 24 hours. As discussed in Chapter 3, glycogen is stored in the muscles and the liver, and the total body store is around 600 g (Murray & Rosenbloom, 2018). Carbohydrate is the fuel used at higher levels of exercise intensity. Even when stores are maximal, each muscle has only a limited amount of glycogen for high-intensity dance, which then needs replacing. It has been estimated that active people can deplete muscle glycogen with 30–60 minutes of high-intensity, intermittent exercise (Coyle, 1995). The amount of glycogen stored in your muscles will have a significant impact on the intensity level you can achieve and sustain in your dance performance. A high muscle glycogen concentration means dancing at your optimal capacity, while low muscle glycogen levels can lead to early fatigue, increased risk of injury and a below-par performance, particularly if the performance includes a significant amount of high-intensity sections. Carbohydrate as glucose and glycogen is the most valuable and important energy-yielding nutrient for dancers. As Impey and colleagues (2018) state: 'the principle of ensuring sufficient carbohydrate (CHO) availability before, during and after training and competition is widely recognized as the fundamental nutritional priority for athletic populations', and dancers can be classed as athletic populations.

A review of the effects of carbohydrate supplementation on exercise performance by Stellingwerff and Cox (2014) who looked at research involving over 650 participants found that over 80% of the 61 studies included showed statistically significant performance benefits, the remaining studies showed no difference to not supplementing. The effects were greater as the duration of the exercise increased. They concluded that there are different mechanisms for carbohydrate benefits depending on the duration of the exercise. When duration is around an hour or less, then there is no benefit from taking carbs from food or drink during the exercise because your body won't have time to digest, absorb and then benefit from the increased carb intake. But, interestingly, using a carb mouth rinse without actually eating any carbs can help, as signals reach the brain from the mouth and this allows enhanced performance. When exercise is longer, two hours or more, then providing extra carbohydrate, up to 90 g or more per hour, to the working muscles for use as fuel enhances performance. The amounts and types of carbohydrate that are useful for dancers will be looked at in more detail shortly.

'Carbs'

Your carbohydrate needs are usually estimated in grams per kilogram of bodyweight (g/kg BW) or grams per hour (g/hr). In dance, as in sport, 'carbs' tends to be shorthand for carbohydrate-rich foods. Most foods identified as a 'carb' will contain other macronutrients and micronutrients but will have these in smaller quantities. Sometimes it is not clear cut, for example, pulses (beans and lentils) are low in fat but provide useful amounts of both carbs and protein, although to get enough of either of these at a meal requires a large portion. Some dancers find it helpful to have an idea of amounts of nutrients, such as carbs and protein, to aim for, as it can be higher than expected. Others find focussing on numbers stressful and prefer to think in more general terms about portion sizes and recommendations for snacks and meals. Both are valid options, whichever works best for you.

II Different types of carbohydrate and their role in the dancer's eating plan

Carbohydrates are classified by their chemical structure, and the most popular method categorises them into two distinct groups: simple (sugars) and complex (starches and fibre). Although carbohydrates are referred to as simple or complex, a simple carbohydrate is not necessarily absorbed quicker, and all carbs have value for dancers.

The terms simple and complex actually refer to the number of sugar molecules in the structure. A single sugar molecule contains carbon (carbo–) as well as oxygen and hydrogen in the same proportion as water (–hydrate). Chemically they are written as $C_X O_{2X} H_X$.

Simple carbohydrates

Simple carbohydrates consist of one- or two-sugar units. **Monosaccharides** are one-sugar units and the most abundant, and most nutritionally important is glucose, a six-carbon sugar written as $C_6 H_{12} O_6$. Fructose, a fruit sugar is also a monosaccharide found in berries, citrus fruits, fruit juice and honey. Galactose, the third main monosaccharide important for many dancers, is found as part of lactose in milk and some other dairy products. **Disaccharides** are formed when two-sugar units are joined together. Sucrose is an example, made up of one glucose unit and one fructose unit bonded together. Commonly known as table sugar, sucrose is obtained from sugar beets or sugar cane. Lactose found in milk is comprised of glucose and galactose. The third main disaccharide in dancers' diets is maltose, formed of two glucose molecules, which is found in sprouted grains, and also when grains are being digested.

Complex carbohydrates

Complex carbohydrates are much larger and **polysaccharides** usually contain hundreds to thousands of sugar units joined together. Starch is a polysaccharide, found in different formats in many plant-based staple foods including rice, pasta, bread and potatoes, as well as cellulose, a non-starch polysaccharide and a type of dietary fibre found in bran, legumes and whole grains. **Oligosaccharides** are found in some vegetables but are also made via food-processing methods. They typically contain around three to ten sugar units. The main oligosaccharides, raffinose and stachyose are found particularly in beans as well as in some vegetables. There are other carbs such as verbascose in this group, all of which can only be digested in the large intestine, by the action of bacteria and with production of gas. Glucose polymers and maltodextrin are oligosaccharides used as bulking agents in processed food as well as sports drinks and meal-replacement products. Figure 4.1 shows the four categories of carbs and the main components of each.

Many foods, either in their natural state or through processing, contain both simple and complex carbohydrates. Flapjacks, for example, contain both complex (oats) and simple (sugar) carbohydrates, and bananas can contain a mixture of sugar and starches depending on their ripeness.

Although a very small amount of carbohydrate can be digested in the mouth and stomach, almost all carbohydrates travel through the digestive tract where the long chains of sugar units are broken down to monosaccharides in the small intestine. The exception is fibre, which is the carbohydrate that cannot be fully broken down by digestive enzymes.

Fibre is crucial to our well-being not only because an adequate fibre intake prevents constipation. The types and amounts of fibre we eat will impact on the balance of bacteria in the large population we have in our large bowel – our microbiome. A low-fibre diet tends to result in less-favourable bacteria being found in increased proportions, and this in turn can impact on health and well-being (Valdes et al., 2018). Although it is possible to take fibre supplements, your best option is to focus on food unless you have a specific medical condition that needs the fibre to be added in a known dose. You can explore what seems best for your body, based around the principles of including at least three portions of veg/salad and two portions of fruit daily, together with wholegrains, beans and lentils, and nuts and seeds in your diet. The area of gut health is explored further in Chapter 13.

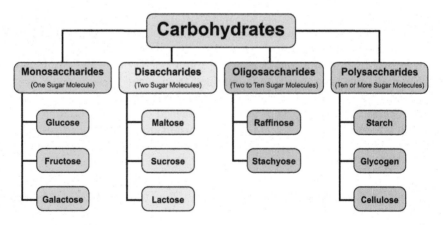

Figure 4.1 Categorisation of carbohydrates.
Credit: Ali DM/Shutterstock.com

III Glycaemic index

Chapter 3 explored the concept in which carbohydrates that are available quickly and impact rapidly on blood glucose levels are known as high glycaemic index (GI) foods, while those where the carbohydrate digestion and absorption are slower are referred to as low GI foods. As with many areas of nutrition, GI is not quite as black and white as it may seem. There are a few points which need to be taken into consideration:

1 When the data are measured, a food is tested on its own, in an amount to provide a standard content of carbohydrate (50 g). This amount may, or may not, relate to normal portion size.
2 Glycaemic load considers the carbohydrate content and the GI together. These data can give a better sense of the likely impact of the food: a tiny piece of cake will have a much smaller impact on blood glucose than a large piece of the same cake.
3 Once sources of protein and/or other types of fibre, for example, vegetables, or fats, or acidic foods are added to the food, this will change (lower) the GI (Flint et al., 2004).

To make it more complicated, there are individual responses to foods. The researchers most experienced in this field acknowledge that this field is difficult but that doesn't mean it should be disregarded (Atkinson et al., 2021). Trying out different foods in combinations, and seeing what seems to be a quick hit, or a slow steady delivery of energy is your best tactic. Make some notes, as different combinations will be useful at different times.

When you have limited time between eating and dance you may find that in fact higher GI foods are preferable to lower: a bean and brown rice salad may leave you feeling uncomfortable, while a chicken or tofu and white rice salad may digest more quickly. If you are about to go on stage for a short intense solo but have been unable to eat recently and are lacking energy, then a bowl of porridge is unlikely to give you that urgent burst of energy, whereas a few jelly babies may help. Planning is always useful, particularly as dance schedules often change, particularly around performances. Meal breaks can end up being shorter than expected, and closer to the performance than expected. Going for higher GI options in these circumstances can help you feel more comfortable and energised for the performance. Table 4.1 gives examples of high and low GI meals.

How do I work out my carbohydrate requirements?

Readers who struggle with a tendency to over focus on the mathematical side of nutrients and nutrient requirements may prefer to bypass the sections on calculating requirements and focus on the qualitative and practical aspects of carbohydrate nutrition.

Table 4.1 Higher and lower GI meal options

Type of meal	Lower GI option	Higher GI option
Hot meal option	Quinoa/basmati rice with protein, e.g., chicken/tofu and vegetables, e.g., peas and broccoli	Mashed potato with protein, e.g., chicken/tofu with vegetables, e.g., courgette, green beans
Cold meal (picnic) option	Wholegrain bread with spread/houmous, protein, e.g., chicken/tofu and salad	Baguette/white bread with spread/houmous, protein, e.g., chicken/tofu and salad

Food rich in carbs is necessary to maintain glucose levels and make sure muscle glycogen stores are kept topped up as far as possible. This food is best eaten regularly over the day, including before, during (if required) and after dance.

The carbohydrate needs of different dance-related exercise are very broad. You may need anywhere from 3 to 4 g of carbohydrate per kilogram of your bodyweight (BW) per day and up to 8–10 g/kg BW per day during long rehearsals or demanding performances (Thomas et al., 2016). The upper level may be even higher under some circumstances. This is due to variations in the duration and intensity of your workload. Dance classes often involve intermittent exercise, with short bursts of anaerobic and aerobic exercise followed by periods of rest (Rodrigues-Krause et al., 2015). This is discussed in more detail in the section on the periodisation of carbohydrate below. The proportions of different intensity activity will drive your carb requirements.

Classes may include skill-based work incorporating some, or all, of the body, complicated balances, small and/or large jumps and steps involving changes of direction and a large use of space. Looking at carbohydrate in terms of requirements per hour, requirements for dance can vary between 30 and 60 g/hr (Baker et al., 2015).

As a general rule, the more of your body you integrate into the dance step (e.g., feet, arms, legs, torso) and the greater the intensity of dance undertaken, the greater your carbohydrate needs will be.

Table 4.2 highlights the different elements of a dance class, rehearsal or performance. A 75-minute ballet class, for example, may involve a 20-minute prior warm-up (comprised of stretching and low-energy movements), 30 minutes at the barre, 25 minutes of centre work, followed by 20 minutes of petit and grand allegro. It will normally include and/or finish with suitable stretching exercises. With a combined time of 95 minutes, a ballet class that slowly increases in intensity could require between 35 and 45 g of carbohydrate/hour.

What does the research say?

There is currently a lack of data on carbohydrate use in different dance genres. This means the best way to estimate carb requirements for different dance genres is to use knowledge of your particular dance genre(s)

Table 4.2 Dance movement types and their classification

Classification of movement type	Description	Example (ballet, contemporary, gym)
Endurance	Continuous activity at varying speeds, often over long distances	Choreographed work (rehearsals, performances on stage), continuous barre or continuous cardio exercise
Power/ strength/high intensity	Frequent short bursts of high-intensity dance, vertically, travelling or with a partner	Grand allegro, e.g., grand jeté, pas de deux (male dancer) Floorwork, flying low technique, virtuosity (jump classes) Resistance training CrossFit
Moderate intensity	Smaller area, short duration	Pirouettes, petit allegro Contemporary techniques, e.g., Cunningham, Graham, Limón and Release
Skill work	Low overall energy demands	Barre and some centre work (e.g., adagio)
Flexibility	Stretches, and exercises that promote flexibility, low-energy demand	Stretching exercises before/during/ after class

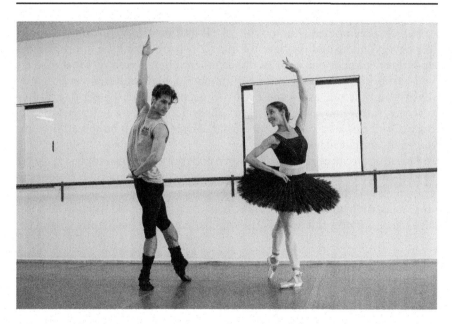

Photo 4.2 Ballet pas de deux include high intensity work which is fuelled by carbohydrate.

Credit: Photo courtesy of Arthur Giglioli

including the range of movements and intensity to adapt the information that is available here to guide you. All styles of dance are characterised by the variety in types of dance movement from less to more intensive, and the duration of different intensity of movement varying. The overall intensity of the workload will drive the requirements for macronutrients, including that from carbohydrate. Intensity of training is often identified by the percentage of maximal heart rate that the exercise requires. You can calculate this roughly by using 220-your age. Once you have an idea of your maximal heart rate you will need to get some information as to what your heart rate is through the class or rehearsal. You can do this by checking your pulse or using data from a heart rate monitor. When using any form of heart rate monitor you are advised to check for accuracy, for example, by taking your pulse as well and seeing how the simultaneous data compare. You can then identify how much of your activity is low intensity, that is where heart rate is around 40–50% of maximal, how much of it is moderate intensity, which is where your heart rate is at approximately 50–75% of your maximum, and how much is high intensity, which is typically defined as exercise at 75% or more of your maximal heart rate.

Recommendations

As you saw above, there are recommendations that suggest for days where all exercise is low intensity or skill based and then 3–5 g carbohydrate/kg body weight is appropriate. It should be noted that 3 g/kg body weight if taken with recommended amounts of fat and protein will result in a very low energy intake and this level of intake is likely to only be appropriate if undertaking under one hour of dance/other activity per day. Most dancers will be working at a combination of moderate, high and even very high intensity, and the ranges for these are 5–7 g carbohydrate/kg per day, 6–10 g carbohydrate/kg/day and 8–12 g carbohydrate/kg body weight/day, respectively. For best-energy levels, your total carb intake will be spread over the day in meals and snacks.

The aim is to meet rather than either under or over consume carbs: in the first instance, your best option is to consider your current intake, your energy levels and the balance of foods that you eat and then consider if changes in your carbohydrate intake might help energy and performance. This is also true for both protein and fats, which are covered in Chapters 5 and 6.

Maximum amounts of carb that can be metabolised per hour

Having an idea of how much carb you need per hour of class/rehearsals/performance is a great starting point. When your activity is more low intensity than high intensity, then the absorption rate of your choice of carb – for example starch, fructose, glucose or maltodextrin – isn't likely to be something that could cause a problem. But if you are working at high intensity for a good proportion of many hours over the day, it may be relevant to pay some attention to this aspect of carb choice.

Typically combinations of carb allow greater absorption than a single source of carb. Much research uses cyclists as participants as it is easy both to standardise and alter the workload. One research study with cyclists in a two-hour exercise trial compared drinking either 8.6% glucose, or the same concentration, but replacing 1/3 of the glucose with fructose and taking 90 g carb/hour, which is a substantial amount during exercise. The mixed carb drink was absorbed more quickly, workload felt easier and heart rates were lower (Jeukendrup & Moseley, 2010). This was a small study, but other studies using combinations of carb sources show similar results because the body is able to benefit from the increased capacity to absorb carbs when the different transport systems for glucose and fructose are used simultaneously. As tolerance is individual, practising is essential before introducing significant amounts of carbs, whether as drinks or solid foods, during breaks in high-intensity dance performances.

Carbohydrate requirements for dance

- The range of amounts given for recommended carbohydrate intakes may seem to be wide, and some dancers may be looking for an exact amount.

- It is important to remember that your activity level varies from day to day, and so your requirements will vary. Although amounts recommended are not precise, they are accurate, and your needs will fall into these ranges.

- An activity diary will help you identify the amount of time you spend working at varying intensity levels, which will allow you to estimate your needs as accurately as possible.

- Remember, you have a great inbuilt system that guides appetite, if you provide your body with a wide range of nutritious foods.

IV Carbohydrate periodisation in dance

The term 'carbohydrate periodisation' is often used to describe the process where carbohydrate availability is manipulated on a day-to-day or even a meal-to-meal basis with most sports research again being in cycling, with as yet, no dance research. It is important to check, when looking at this research for potential application to dance. For example, whether it is just the timing of carbohydrate within the day that varies, and overall carbohydrate intake will be adequate, meeting requirements, or on the other hand, whether carbohydrate periodisation is a process of being in a carbohydrate deficit, so it is both controlled for timing and to be at a level below requirements. Clearly, this is a very different situation, as choosing to deliberately underfuel is something you are likely to find unhelpful to both your dance performance and your health.

What does the research say?

While there are data in sport on this concept of periodisation, frequently research is undertaken as a single event rather than sequentially, or at most, looking at two training sessions per day. One strategy for the periodisation of CHO availability used in sport would be limiting carbohydrate intake after glycogen-depleting intensive interval training and then training less intensively with limited glycogen stores the following day. This is possible when training for a sport where there are clearly identified times of lower and higher intensity training, and this can be controlled by the athlete. Dance does not have usually have these clear distinctions, and every class, rehearsal and performance will include a mixture of lower and higher-intensity activity, which is rarely under the dancer's control.

Marquet et al. (2016) have reported that a week of well-fueled afternoon training sessions followed by limited carbohydrate intake, then a training session the following morning with reduced glycogen stores leads to an up-regulation of several exercise-responsive signalling proteins in their study using 11 well-trained male endurance cyclists. The authors stated that:

> Implementing the "sleep-low" strategy (whereby athletes complete training but do not fully refuel for the work done) for one-week improved performance by the same magnitude previously seen in a three-week intervention, without any significant changes in selected markers of metabolism.

It is necessary to remember that these are male endurance cyclists, all aiming to consume 6 g carb/kg body weight per day (which is a moderate level for active people), and the low carbohydrate training was low-intensity cycling at 65% of maximal heart rate. Performance in a 20 km time trail cycling race at the end of the training week improved in the 'sleep-low' group compared with the more normally distributed carbohydrate group. This is interesting, but the participant numbers are small and although not statistically significant the train low group had a higher energy and carbohydrate intake compared with the control group. One participant had a very dramatic increase in performance which will have impacted on the results, and larger studies are needed to evaluate whether the results would be replicated.

Impey et al. (2018) state that "deliberately training with reduced CHO availability to enhance endurance-training-induced metabolic adaptations of skeletal muscle (i.e., the 'train low, compete high' paradigm) is a hot topic within sport nutrition. Train-low studies involve periodically training (e.g., 30–50% of training sessions) with reduced CHO availability, where train-low models include twice per day training, fasted training, post-exercise CHO restriction and 'sleep low, train low'".

Conclusions

Conclusions from this area of research are that participants' work capacity during exercise is something which must be taken into consideration.

When athletes have been in a low carbohydrate state, they cannot exercise as intensively. Clearly, for dancers with limited time to learn and perform, struggling with energy levels is not optimal. In fact, Impey et al. concluded when considering performance rather than biochemical changes in the body: 'nonetheless, such muscle adaptations do not always translate to improved exercise performance, for example, 37% and 63% of 11 studies show improvements or no change, respectively'. They propose a concept of glycogen threshold which is the level of muscle glycogen concentration is enough to allow athletes/dancers to successfully complete their physical workload but also becomes depleted during the training sessions to achieve the best physiological training adaptations to make the workload less tiring in the future. This needs much more research to quantify how this could be used for athletes and dancers, but the future may bring developments which may help your performance.

Estimating for energy demands

Impey and colleagues (2018) suggest that athletes – which current thinking would include dancers – 'fuel for the work required' whereby CHO availability is adjusted in accordance with the demands of the upcoming training session(s). This strategy proposes that athletes plan their intake in advance of their training sessions. They suggest that the long-term goal of research is to 'ensure absolute training intensity is not compromised, while also creating a metabolic milieu conducive to facilitating the endurance phenotype', in other words to try and have a metabolism that uses carbohydrate as efficiently as possible while also having a body that is appropriately fuelled for the demands of the physical workload.

To try and estimate carbohydrate requirements in advance is much harder for dancers than for sports people. In the current dance training and performance model, dancers in full-time training and those working professionally are likely to be working with a number of teachers, choreographers, etc., rather than just one coach, and planning the intensity of training over a day/week is still a concept in its early stages. As there are clear concerns that dancers are at risk of under-fuelling (Keay et al., 2020), for the present, dancers are advised where possible to listen to their body which will signal if insufficient food has been received and attempt to drive an intake to respond to this, while also using knowledge to plan as far as possible for the likely intensity of the day's work.

As well as taking enough carbs, consuming enough protein and fat as well will allow dancers to meet their energy needs and be best prepared to approach their workload with energy.

How to spread your carbs out over the day

Using the information above you can, if you wish, get an idea of your total carbohydrate needs whether estimated from the daily requirement for body weight, or the hourly guidelines for exercise intensity. Your total is likely to be somewhere between 250 and 500 g carb/day, depending on your body size and workload. There will be a small number of dancers who need a little less, although 200 g/day is likely to be the lowest usual requirement. A few with very high requirements may need more than this range, but it will cover many dancers' needs. These figures are given so that when you look at the tables with portions of carbohydrate, you have some context and thought about how this comes together into a meal plan that best meets your needs.

Typically the main carb items in a meal need to give you 50–100 g, with snacks being anywhere from 10 g upwards (a piece of fruit), though snacks around 20–40 g carb will be more useful to most dancers. Those with high requirements may find it works best to have three meals and three snacks, with one of these snacks being substantial – e.g., porridge/cereal with additions, similar to breakfast.

Some examples of snacks to provide 20–30 g carb are provided in Table 4.3.

A quick note on cereal and other bars

Bars can be very useful, but not all bars are the same nutritionally. Apart from differences in size/weight, which of course impact on the nutrient content, the ingredients can vary hugely. There is no right or wrong here, the aim is to select a bar which meets your needs for the time you need the snack. A bar where sugar and versions of sugar (sucrose/glucose/fructose) are the main ingredients or are listed as the second or third ingredient is likely to offer less in the way of nutrients other than carb compared to a bar where a grain (oats, wheat), dried fruit, nuts or seeds are main ingredients, which will provide some protein, vitamins and minerals. Check where oils/fats are in the list too – for quick digestion you want to avoid the higher-fat bars.

Looking at the nutritional content, if the carb:fat ratio is at least 3:1, for example, 27 g carb and 7 g fat or 37 g carb and 6 g fat, the ratio is good for active refuelling. Bars where the amount of fat is closer to the amount of carb, for example, 26 g carb and 11 g fat, the ratio isn't so good for meeting your targets for enough carbs. This can be worked round by having some extra fruit or dried fruit with higher-fat bars.

Sugar cravings

- Carbohydrate is needed for many processes in life, and for high-intensity dance work.

- Carbohydrate cravings can occur for many reasons, but inadequate intake of carbohydrates can be the cause for many dancers.

- Lack of sleep, fluid and other nutrients may also be the cause.

- Hormonal fluctuations can contribute.

- There may be more than one reason at any one time.

Table 4.3 Snacks: each provides 20–30 g carb

Snacks to each provide 20–30 g carb

Cereal bar – see notes	Fruit yoghurt: individual pot with 1 tbsp raisins	One slice/55 g banana bread (or other fruit bread)	Four rice cakes, plain or with topping of choice	Malt loaf – two slices (or two mini loaves)
Large banana (190 g with skin)	Soya fruit yoghurt with 2 tbsp raisins	Six to seven breadsticks with salsa or similar dip	Mini-pitta with hoummous and raw veg	Small fruit scone with jam
One slice bread/toast with jam/ honey	four rich tea biscuits	One Weetabix/ Wheat Bisks/wheat biscuits or oat biscuits with milk and berries	One oatcakes plain or with topping of choice	Fruit smoothie: two portions of fruit with milk/ yoghurt of choice
30 g pretzels	Two to three Digestive biscuits	Two scotch pancakes	125–150 g natural yoghurt with fresh or dried fruit	Small fruit flapjack (about 40 g)
½ bagel with jam or honey	Small bowl cereal with milk	Four to five dates	1/2 hot cross/fruit bun and jam	½ a tortilla wrap spread with applesauce or peanut butter (roll up and cut into slices)

Table 4.4 gives approximate portion sizes to provide either 50 or 80 g carbohydrate from one type of food, using household measures, for comparison where possible. Because meals can vary in their carb content, and many people would, for example, be used to eating more carb from pasta than bread, some amounts might look more or less appropriate to you. This guide can help you to find the easiest way to meet your needs on days when more carbs are needed. And, of course, you can combine different foods which can make the meal more interesting. If you need more precise information, it's best to use the information on the packaging, or from a nutrition database, or speak to a qualified dietitian or nutritionist. Although you may see information that vegetables provide carbs, in reality the amount of carb from a portion of most vegetables will be less than 5 g. Even vegetables often regarded as more starchy, such as carrots, pumpkin, swede and turnip, will only provide a maximum of 10 g carb per portion. Sweetcorn,

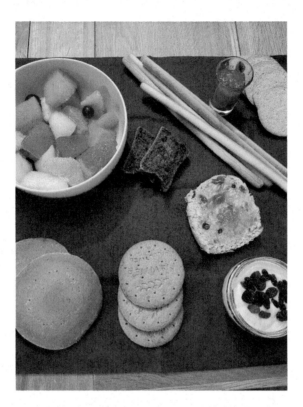

Photo 4.3 Carbohydrate rich snacks.

beetroot and butternut squash are a little higher and including one of these in meals can be a useful way to top up carb intakes, as a portion of either will provide 10–15 g carb. You can see the very large amount of beetroot needed for 50 g carb in Table 4.5. You will also see that only potatoes, sweet potato, parsnip and yam are included as starchy vegetables which can provide us with significant amounts of carb. While pulses (beans and lentils) are a useful source of protein and carb, to rely on pulses to meet your carb goals will mean eating very bulky meals, so they are best used in combination with another carb source.

V The role of carbohydrate in recovery from exercise, including dance

There is now a substantial amount of data from sport that carbohydrate re-fuelling is best started as soon as possible after activity (Jentjens & Jeukendrup, 2003). The longer the gap between intense exercise and taking in some carbs, whether in food or drink, the longer the refuelling process will take. Getting some carb-rich food into your body within an hour of finishing exercise is best. Ninety minutes is the longest gap you should leave between dance and eating if you don't want to delay your glycogen recovery. This is

Table 4.4 Carbs for meals: some are best used in combinations

Food portion for 50 g carb	Food portion for 50 g carb	Food portion for 50 g carb	Food portion for 80 g carb	Food portion for 80 g carb	Food portion for 80 g carb
Five egg-sized boiled potatoes	Basmati rice, 1/3 cup before cooking	75 g uncooked pasta	Eight egg-sized boiled potatoes	Basmati rice ½ cup before cooking	110 g uncooked pasta
2½-thick slices bread	Couscous, cooked: one cup	Quinoa: 260 g cooked weight	Four thick slices bread	Couscous, cooked: 1½ cups	Quinoa: 415 g cooked weight
Noodles 1.2 blocks/nests (about 180 g cooked)	One cup oats (uncooked)	One very large or two medium baked sweet potatoes	Noodles two portions/blocks (about 290 g cooked)	1½-cup oats (uncooked weight)	Two large sweet potatoes
Mashed potato: Two rounded serving spoons	One large Jacket potato	165 g cooked potato wedges	Mashed potato: three rounded serving spoons	Two medium Jacket potato	260 g cooked potato wedges
One large wrap	One large pitta bread	320 g cooked polenta	1½ large wraps	Two medium pitta bread	500 g cooked polenta
Butter beans 380 g cooked weight (about 1½ cans)	Red lentils (cooked): 285 g	Beetroot: 500 g	Butter beans 610 g cooked weight (about 2½ cans)	Red lentils (cooked): 460 g	Beetroot: 800 g
Parsnip, boiled: 390 g	Pearl barley: 400 g cooked weight	150g boiled yam (2½ medium slices)	Parsnip, boiled: 620 g	Pearl barley: 640 g cooked weight	240 g boiled yam (four medium slices)

not new data, and some elite dancers have followed this advice over recent years. But dancers face challenges to this. Often after a performance, there is a focus on practical tasks, such as getting costumes stored and stage make up removed. Also, appetite is often not good at this point. As ex-ballerina Deborah Bull neatly put it, 'the most important time to eat, perhaps para-doxically, is the time you least feel like it: after the show' (Bull, 2011).

Consuming around 1 g per kg body weight carbohydrate, soon after dance will start the refuelling process. This is not additional carbohydrate but comes from your daily total so there is no need to try and get all your

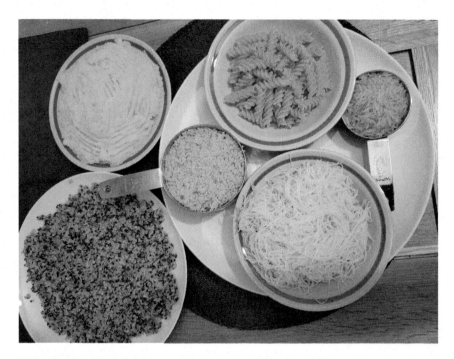

Photo 4.4 Portions of foods each to provide approx. 50g carb.

carbs in before a performance. Planning for a meal or snack that you can have within 30 minutes of coming off stage is a great strategy. This means prioritising refuelling. Thinking about what you find most palatable after a show is a good starting point, and also what is practical, e.g., if you need to bring food with you to the venue. It is not essential to aim for high-fibre foods after performances and intense training, as the aim is for quick availability not slow delivery to the muscles. Table 4.5 gives some suggestions.

VI A note about carbohydrate intake when injured

Your nutritional requirements after an injury, and whether these are different to your normal requirements, will depend completely on what the injury is, what the treatment is and how much it impacts on your ability to complete your normal dance and activity schedule.

If you have an injury that doesn't have a significant impact on your dance schedule and overall activity levels, then it is unlikely that you need to alter your carb intake.

If you have to reduce activity, then if possible go with your appetite to make adjustments to your intake – or use the guides given in this chapter.

Table 4.5 Post-performance refuelling options

Preferred option after performances	*Suggestions for carb refuelling*
Main meal – as only light meals eaten in the day/higher requirements	1. Pasta with tomato sauce. Include protein too if needed, low-fat choices such as chicken/fish/lentils are best 2. Rice or noodles with vegetables and chicken/tofu 3. Sweet potato and veg stew with chicken/Quorn
Light meal as main meal taken earlier in the day	1. Baked beans on toast with fruit/yoghurt 2. A wrap with chicken/beans and salad. Fruit/yoghurt 3. Jacket potato with beans/tuna and veg/salad
Snack as both a main meal and light meal was eaten before performance	1. A bowl of cereal with milk and fruit 2. Soup and bread/crackers 3. Yoghurt with fruit and muesli

If you are in pain, this can impact on your appetite and result in possibly eating less than you need: be mindful of this as you may have to treat food more as part of your treatment if your appetite drops. If you have to have any surgery, then there will most likely be time that you can't eat, so making sure you don't under-eat before or after the surgery is important for recovery.

In rehab from injuries, carbs are still an essential part of a well-balanced dancer's diet, regardless of how much dance they do. Carb-rich foods such as oats, grains, beans, lentils, fruits and starchy vegetables provide many other useful nutrients as well as energy. If your rehab process is intense, or your injury requires you to use crutches, your energy needs may in fact be comparable to your lower-intensity dance days.

VII Low carbohydrate diets and their impact on dance performance

As dance involves high-intensity activity, for classes, rehearsals and performance, which is fuelled by carbs, a low-carb diet isn't likely to lead to good energy levels for the high-intensity work. A low carbohydrate diet is unlikely to leave you able to perform at your best, unless the dance you are undertaking is low intensity only. You may have seen information about low-carb training in sport where research on how/whether it is possible to manipulate the type of fuel – fat or carbs – used by the body is ongoing. It seems that in endurance events, such marathons or ultra-marathons, there can be some adaptations, but dancers do not work constantly at the same pace, below high intensity, for long periods of time (Rauch et al., 2021). However, it is always useful to check on research updates from both sport and dance nutrition from time to time as useful updates and strategies can emerge.

The risk of low energy availability on a low-carb diet

Think about your overall intake – protein and fats together with carbs. A low-carb diet is going to mean a higher intake of fat and/or protein. If you are not managing to take in enough energy, from these combined then rather than being in a low-carb but adequate energy state, you are in a low-energy state and at risk of RED-S which is discussed in Chapter 11. Louise Burke, an eminent Australian sports dietitian, and her colleagues researched whether athletes meet their carb targets and concluded that it was likely most male athletes did. Female athletes were more at risk of not doing so, particularly if they felt under pressure to achieve or maintain low levels of body fat. But she concludes that 'what is known for certain is that increased carb availability enhances endurance and performance during single exercise sessions' (Burke et al., 2001). As dancers have at least one exercise session per day, whether it be a performance (or two), rehearsals or classes – or a combination of these – taking in enough carbohydrate is a way to support both stamina and technique.

VIII Resources

Carbohydrates – The Master Fuel|U.S. Anti-Doping Agency (USADA).
High-Quality Carbohydrates and Physical Performance – PMC (nih.gov).
Glycaemic Index Food Fact Sheet|British Dietetic Association (BDA).
'Carbs and cals' App: an app (small cost) originally designed for those with diabetes, this app has photos of different portions of foods and their carb (and other macronutrient) content.

IX Learning outcomes

After reading this chapter the reader should be able to:

1   Describe different types of carbohydrates and foods in which they are found.
2   Discuss the best times to eat low and high GI foods.
3   Explain the potential consequences of a low carbohydrate diet on a dancer's performance.
4   Suggest some suitable meals for dancers after performances.

References

Atkinson, F.S. et al. (2021) International tables of glycemic index and glycemic load values 2021: A systematic review, *The American Journal of Clinical Nutrition,* 114(5), pp.1625–1632.

Baker, L.B. et al. (2015) Acute effects of carbohydrate supplementation on intermittent sports performance, *Nutrients,* 7(7), pp.5733–5763.

Bull, D. (2011) *The Everyday Dancer,* Faber & Faber, London, p.72.

Burke, L.M. (2001) Guidelines for daily carbohydrate intake: Do athletes achieve them? *Sports Medicine,* 31(4), pp.267–299.

Coyle, E.F. (1995) Substrate utilization during exercise in active people, *The American Journal of Clinical Nutrition,* 61(4), pp.968S–979S.

Flint, A. et al. (2004) The use of glycaemic index tables to predict glycaemic index of composite breakfast meals, *British Journal of Nutrition,* 91(6), pp.979–989.

Impey, S.G. et al. (2018) Fuel for the work required: A theoretical framework for carbohydrate periodization and the glycogen threshold hypothesis, *Sports Medicine,* 48(5), pp.1031–1048.

Jentjens, R. and Jeukendrup, A.E. (2003) Determinants of post-exercise glycogen synthesis during short-term recovery, *Sports Medicine,* 33(2), pp.117–144.

Jeukendrup, A.E. and Moseley, L. (2010) Multiple transportable carbohydrates enhance gastric emptying and fluid delivery, *Scandinavian Journal of Medicine & Science in Sports,* 20(1), pp.112–121.

Keay, N., Overseas, A. and Francis, G. (2020) Indicators and correlates of low energy availability in male and female dancers, *BMJ Open Sport & Exercise Medicine,* 6(1), pp.e000906.

Marquet, L. et al. (2016) Periodization of carbohydrate intake: Short-term effect on performance, *Nutrients,* 8(12), p.755.

Murray, B. and Rosenbloom, C. (2018) Fundamentals of glycogen metabolism for coaches and athletes, *Nutrition Reviews,* 76(4), pp.243–259.

Rauch, C.E. et al. (2021) Feeding tolerance, glucose availability, and whole-body total carbohydrate and fat oxidation in male endurance and ultra-endurance runners in response to prolonged exercise, consuming a habitual mixed macronutrient diet and carbohydrate feeding during exercise. *Frontiers in Physiology,* 12, pp.773054.

Rodrigues-Krause, J., Krause, M. and Reischak-Oliveira, Á. (2015) Cardiorespiratory considerations in dance: From classes to performances, *Journal of Dance Medicine & Science,* 19(3), pp.91–102.

Stellingwerff, T. and Cox, G.R. (2014) Systematic review: Carbohydrate supplementation on exercise performance or capacity of varying durations, *Applied Physiology, Nutrition, and Metabolism,* 39(9), pp.998–1011.

Thomas, D.T., Erdman, K.A. and Burke, L.M. (2016) Position of the academy of nutrition and dietetics, dietitians of Canada, and the American college of sports medicine: Nutrition and athletic performance, *Journal of the Academy of Nutrition and Dietetics,* 116(3), pp.501–528.

Valdes, A.M. et al. (2018) Role of the gut microbiota in nutrition and health, *British Medical Journal,* 361, pp.36–44.

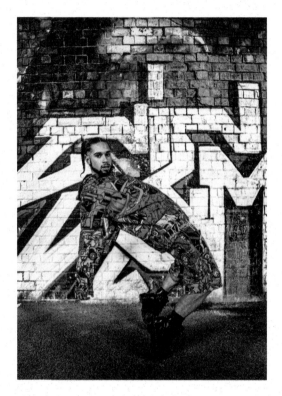

Photo 5.1 Protein is essential for dancers to remain strong and healthy.
Source: Photo courtesy of Dani Bower photography

5 Protein for strength and body maintenance

Contents

Protein myths	Reality
More protein will result in bulky muscles.	Muscle growth is the result of particular types of training combined with diet.
Gaining strength will result in bulky muscles.	Muscle size is not directly linked to muscle strength: the type of training will determine this.
Eating a normal protein intake but low fat/carb will not compromise strength.	When energy intake is low, there is a risk that protein will be used for energy and that muscles will be broken down.
After injury nutrition requirements are lower.	Nutrient requirements after injury can be very variable: an increase in protein intake is likely to be beneficial for many dancers.

I A dancer's protein requirements

Introduction to protein

As you saw in Chapter 3, the term 'protein' covers a range of different molecules with different structures. They all have the common components of amino acids made from carbon, hydrogen, oxygen and nitrogen, sometimes

DOI: 10.4324/9781003219002-5

with sulphur. The name amino acid comes from the fact that amino acids include an amino group ($-NH_2$) and a carboxylic acid group ($-COOH$). Proteins are found in most foods, but often at levels where it would not be possible to get all your protein from those foods due to the bulk – for example, vegetables and fruits – where you would typically need several kilos per day.

There is an interaction between protein and exercise, in that dancers need adequate protein to gain benefit from training. Sports nutrition research has focussed on the amounts of protein needed by different groups of athletes, as well as the type of protein and the timing of protein intake with respect to training sessions. This can be adapted for dance, as each of these areas is useful to explore to allow you to dance at your best.

The many roles of protein in the body

When thinking about protein requirements for the body, most people will focus on the need for protein for muscle growth and repair. This is indeed a key role of protein for a dancer, but there are many other essential roles that protein plays in your body. These include:

i **Structural components: muscles, bones, tendons and ligaments**
Protein is needed for muscles; however, protein alone does not increase muscle strength or size. It is the combination of physical workload and nutrition that is needed for muscles to gain strength. Significant muscle growth will not take place without substantial physical workload above and beyond that normally undertaken together with an adequate protein intake. Details on amounts for this are given in Section III. While there is a correlation between muscle strength and muscle size, there are several other factors that are involved in this relationship, including the workload, (specifically intensity), how specific the training is and the frequency of training (Morton et al., 2019; Reggiani & Schiaffino, 2020).
Repair:
Collagen, a major component of bone, is protein. Collagen is also needed for skin, muscles, tendons, ligaments and cartilage, so protein is needed in the repair processes from day-to-day wear and tear as well as after injury.
Hair, which has some protective functions for the body, is also made predominantly from protein.

ii **Transport**
Protein has a role in transporting nutrients and oxygen within the body. Lipoproteins are responsible for transporting fats and cholesterol within the body. Haemoglobin, in red blood cells, is the molecule which transports oxygen from the lungs to all cells in the body. A low-protein diet has been shown to result in a drop in haemoglobin (Shiraki et al.,

1977). Protein has also been shown to be essential for the formation of red blood cells (Deen et al., 2021, which are crucial to the transport of carbon dioxide from the cells back to the lungs where it can be expired. Because red blood cells are responsible for delivering oxygen to working muscles, dancers not getting sufficient protein may become fatigued during activity. Protein is therefore essential for a well-functioning cardiorespiratory system.

iii **Enzymes**

There are thousands of enzymes, made of protein, in the body. Enzymes are needed to allow the many chemical reactions in your body to take place. They play a vital role without being altered at the end of the process (Lewis & Stone 2020). You may be familiar with enzymes involved in digestion, such as amylase, needed for carbohydrate breakdown, while lipase and protease are involved in fat and protein breakdown. There are many other enzymes dancers are dependent on, such as creatine kinase needed for the formation of phosphocreatine, which was discussed in Chapter 3. Dancer's not getting enough protein may find they have reduced power, which would affect their jump height and their capacity to lift a partner.

iv **The immune system**

Protein has a major role in the effective working of the immune system. White blood cells, made in your bone marrow, produce antibodies and proteins which fight foreign substances within the body. A healthy immune system minimises time lost due to illness.

v **Other functions of protein**

Some hormones are proteins.

Protein is needed to maintain the balance of acids and alkalis, as well as fluids, in the body.

Protein is needed for the nervous system as a component of neurotransmitters, essential for many technical elements of dance, such as fast reaction times, proprioception and alignment.

Protein as a source of energy

As discussed previously, in Chapter 3, protein can be used as a source of energy, but if energy intake is low and protein needs to be used for energy, then it is not available for all the functions described above.

Protein turnover

As a dancer, you need more protein than less active people, so that your body is able to respond to the demands of training by building and sustaining strength, as well as maintaining normal body functions. There is an ongoing process of muscle breakdown and muscle repair occurring in the muscles. This process, which results in protein turnover, will be increased when physical activity – such as dance – is undertaken more intensively than for the general population. Research shows that it can take 24 hours after resistance exercise is undertaken before the rates of protein turnover (both synthesis and breakdown) return to pre-exercise levels (Biolo, 1995). In dance training when muscles undertake strenuous work, the fibres within them can become damaged and will need protein for repair. The dance workload is frequently designed to stimulate muscle synthesis, by the use of resistance rather than endurance activities, which will require additional protein over and above that needed by less active people.

Protein and muscle protein synthesis

Research shows that the way in which the body responds to protein being ingested straight after exercise depends on a number of factors. When you begin new or unfamiliar training your muscles respond differently to additional protein compared with repeating familiar training. When you undertake an unfamiliar workload, muscles are slower to respond by increasing muscle protein synthesis (MPS) but respond more and for longer, and there is more

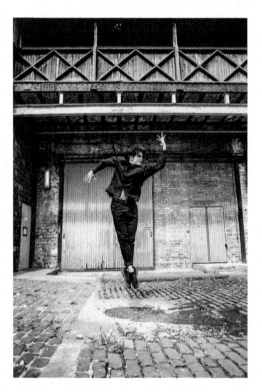

Photo 5.2 Protein is necessary for dancers' strength and performance.
Source: Photo courtesy of Dani Bower photography

muscle damage which needs repair before muscle growth takes priority. The type (for example, eccentric versus concentric exercise), frequency and duration of resistance training will likely all result in differences, and often studies are done with small numbers of participants. There are also some challenges in the methodology which make it hard to interpret data. In dance, the training is not consistent from one session to another, and the workload will be adapted to allow the progression of technique. This means that studying how dancers can best use nutrition to support strength gain is challenging, but what is very clear is that adequate protein together with appropriate training is vital for the dancer to gain the necessary strength. This strength gain may need to be addressed outside of class if class is focussing only on technique rather than also optimising physiological capacity to do the work.

Dancers wishing to explore the mechanisms of MPS in more detail are encouraged to look at the paper by Hodson et al. (2019).

II Essential and non-essential amino acids

To recap the information in Chapter 3, protein is made up of amino acids which contain carbon, hydrogen and oxygen with the addition of nitrogen, and in some cases, sulphur.

Peptide bonds join amino acids together into peptide chains of 2–50 amino acids and proteins of over 50 amino acids.

There are 21 amino acids used by humans, nine of which are described as 'essential amino acids' (EAA) or 'indispensable amino acids'. The nine EEA must be obtained from food. Six of the non-EEA have been identified as conditionally essential/indispensable where they become essential in specific situations such as when the body has experienced stress during growth or after trauma. More research is needed to clarify when each may become essential and when the body can synthesise them. The final six amino acids can always be synthesised within the body; however, all 21 are essential for your body to function. Table 5.1 shows the 21 amino acids you need.

In terms of nutrition, a food with all nine EAA is known as a 'complete protein'. A food which contains protein, but not all nine EAA, is known as an 'incomplete protein'. Plant-based foods are more likely to be incomplete proteins, which has implications when thinking about the amount of protein that is needed each day.

There can also be low levels of one or more EAA in foods, which will have an impact on how well the protein can be used. For example, grains tend to be low in lysine, while beans and lentils are low in methionine. Combining foods in meals is a globally accepted method as being the best way to allow your body to make the best use of the protein content, for example, a bean or lentil dish with rice or bread. The term used to describe when the EAA in an incomplete protein is low compared to the level seen in complete proteins is 'limiting amino acid'.

Table 5.1 Amino acids

Amino acids		
Essential/indispensable amino acids	*Conditionally essential/ indispensable amino acids*	*Non-essential/non-indispensable amino acids*
Phenylalanine	Glutamine	Alanine
Valine	Proline	Serine (sometimes considered conditionally essential)
Tryptophan	Tyrosine	Asparagine
Threonine	Glycine	Aspartic Acid
Isoleucine	Cysteine	Glutamic Acid
Methionine	Arginine	Selenocysteine (recently identified so not always included in the list of amino acids needed by humans)
Histidine		
Leucine		
Lysine		

Each amino acid has a unique side chain which impacts the structure proteins will form when amino acids are joined together and this will impact on the function of the protein. When protein in food is digested and eventually broken down into amino acids, the combinations of amino acids with different side chains are relevant in the rebuilding process, for example to create muscle, ligaments or tendons. For this all to occur effectively in your body, an adequate intake of all EAA and a total protein intake to meet your needs are required.

Amino acids containing sulphur or selenium

Methionine and cysteine both contain sulphur, while selenocysteine contains selenium rather than sulphur. Selenomethionine is a form of methionine found in food, for example, Brazil nuts, which contains selenium. Selenocysteine is the form of cysteine containing selenium. Selenium-containing amino acids can act as antioxidants within the body. This can be as direct action, or by acting as a source of selenium for the production of antioxidants (Rahmanto & Davies, 2012). For more information on why you need selenium see Appendix A.

Branched-chain amino acids

Leucine, isoleucine and valine are known as the branched-chain amino acids (BCAA) due to their structure. BCAA are found in beef, chicken, fish, eggs, milk and soy. Beans, lentils and chickpeas are good plant-based sources.

There is some evidence that BCAA supplements may help stimulate MPS after resistance exercise (Jackman et al., 2017), but it is most likely that the effect of BCAA on MPS is due to the leucine content rather than the combination of the three amino acids (Witard et al., 2019), and dancers are therefore advised to focus on leucine.

Leucine

There is evidence that dancers can and do benefit from the major role that leucine has in initiating MPS. In one study, dancers who took a supplement of whey protein, which has a high leucine content, noted accelerated recovery following acute exercise-induced muscle damage (Brown et al., 2018). If you are using plant-based milk alternatives, then you will need to consume more to achieve the same intake of leucine, compared to whey protein. Soy protein has around 80% of the leucine content of whey protein (Norton et al., 2012). Pea, brown rice protein, corn and potato supplements have a satisfactory amount of EAA compared with the overall protein content. Each of these also contains a satisfactory amount of leucine. Other plant protein alternatives, such as oat and hemp, have low EAA as a percentage of the total protein and will also have low leucine contents (Gorissen et al., 2018).

As well as supporting MPS when combined with resistance exercise, leucine is recognised as decreasing central nervous system fatigue which can occur in endurance exercise and result in reduced performance as the body attempts to reduce the risk of damage. There doesn't seem to be an increase in injury risk when using protein to decrease central nervous system fatigue and reduce the perceived workload (Newsholme & Blomstrand, 2006), but dancers are advised to be mindful of their workload and take adequate rest, rather than using decreased fatigue to work longer/harder.

Leucine and the older dancer

Maintaining muscle mass becomes harder after the age of 30: it is estimated that muscle mass decreases approximately 3–8% per decade after the age of 30. This rate of decline is even higher after the age of 60 (Volpi et al., 2004). For the dancer wishing to maintain muscle mass, taking on adequate protein that is leucine rich in combination with undertaking resistance exercise, becomes even more important from age 30 onwards. Meals that contain 30–40 g of protein have been shown to be beneficial for MPS in older adults (Witard et al., 2016), and an increased intake of leucine can mitigate the effects of ageing on MPS (Devries et al., 2018). Those on highly plant-based diet are advised to focus on protein-rich foods which have a good leucine content, as there is evidence that a minimum 'dose' of 3 g leucine (from food or a supplement) is needed for it to have an impact on MPS (Zaromskyte et al., 2021). There is a need for more studies on females, as most research has used male participants, but until data is available female dancers are advised to use the above recommendations.

Leucine

Leucine is a key amino acid which has a specific role in protein metabolism: it seems to be the 'dimmer switch' which turns on protein repair and creation in muscles according to the amount you take in up to a maximal dose. Response to leucine appears to be more sensitive in young dancers than older dancers, so older dancers may benefit from a higher intake of protein rich in leucine.

Dancers who supplemented with whey protein, which is high in leucine, have observed accelerated recovery following acute exercise-induced muscle damage.

III Dietary protein and goal setting

Introduction

Dancers' protein goals for are, as for athletes, higher than for the general population. This section looks at the factors that can impact your individual requirements, which will also change from time to time as your workload and dance goals change. Theory into practice – information on specific foods – is covered later in the chapter.

The dietary reference value (DRV) for protein intake in the UK is the amount estimated to be enough for 97% of the general population group. For the general population aged 19–64 years, the DRV is currently 0.75 g protein per kg body weight per day. This has been translated as 45 g for females per day and 55.5 g for males. The figures for those aged 15–18 years are 45 g for females and 55.2 g for males. There is no consideration in these figures for those who are more active and might have a higher protein need to maintain muscle mass.

Protein goals for dancers

From the sports world until recently, advice for endurance athletes was to take in not less than 1.2 g per kg bodyweight (BW) per day of protein (1.2 g protein/kg/day). Strength athletes would aim for a higher level, around 1. 6–2 g protein/kg/day. This has been updated and slightly modified to advise athletes to take 1.2–2 g protein/kg/day depending on workload and goals within a periodised training programme. Short term intakes can even be higher for specific goals: the upper limit of recommended intake is now around 2.5 g protein/kg/day (Thomas et al., 2016).

As dancers' workloads are often unpredictable, an average of around 1.6 g protein/kg/day represents a level that is likely to meet your requirements without being excessive. It isn't helpful either financially or environmentally to overdo protein and it can impact health if consumed at extremely high levels. If there is a specific goal for strength gain then it may be appropriate to aim for 2 g protein/kg/day until that goal is reached. For those who personally feel that looking at numbers is unhelpful and can result in over focus on food, it is not necessary to know exactly what your weight is, nor to be over-precise in calculations: the aim is to have an idea of levels of protein that will best support your dance workload, and to understand this will, in any case be variable. While protein can't be stored, the human body is able to tolerate variations in intake, and having a general understanding of a minimum requirement and an approximate goal will be useful.

While much of the research has been done in males, until female-specific advice is available it would seem best to follow the current consensus. In particular, it is good practice that you include meals or snacks containing both carbohydrate and protein relatively speedily after exercise to help maintain muscle and promote glycogen restoration. Timing is much less crucial for protein than for carb refuelling, but to meet your requirements it makes sense to include protein regularly. See Section IV for information on timing.

Are some protein sources better than others?

High-quality protein is the focus, whether this is from a single source or by planned combinations. High quality for dancers means complete proteins, which includes meat, poultry, fish, eggs, Quorn, milk, cheese, yoghurt and soy. Pulses, nuts or seeds combined with grains together provide a complete protein profile. Quinoa is a complete protein, but, as with many plant proteins, a relatively large portion will be needed to meet the meal protein targets for many dancers.

Protein for different dance styles

Although there is currently a lack of research on protein requirements for different dance genres, consideration of different movement types, the requirement for additional strength for specific choreography and workload can guide you towards the best estimate of your protein goals. This can work across dance genres, as within a genre the workload can vary considerably. If you are unsure, then the guide of 1.6 g protein/kg/day is likely to be adequate, unless you specifically need to build muscle for a piece with more lifts or upper body work than usual. Following a break, for example, a dance student's summer holidays, or a company member's off season, as you prepare for the new term/season, particularly if you are focussing on gaining strength, aiming closer to 2 g protein/kg/day would be useful. While muscle can respond quickly to appropriate strength training, many studies use 4–12 week periods to evaluate outcomes, so allowing at least four weeks to see useful progress is suggested.

Fine-tuning protein goals

Having identified your protein needs for your schedule, there are a number of additional factors and situations that can impact on a dancer's protein requirements and should also be considered. Some, none, or all of these may apply at different times, meaning that it is helpful to review how well you are meeting your needs when your personal situation changes. Asking yourself the following questions will guide you towards more individualised protein goals:

1   Are you a vegetarian or vegan dancer?
    Vegetarians and vegans are likely to benefit from increasing their protein intake slightly above the amounts advised above. One reason is that many vegetarian sources of protein, for example, beans and lentils and nuts and seeds, do not contain all the EAA. Protein combining, the advice to complement proteins low in different amino acids within a meal is not essential, but the general concept to ensure varied protein over a day is still useful for all vegetarians/vegans. A practical example, which features naturally in many food plans is to combine lentils or beans (low in methionine) with rice or wheat (low in lysine, threonine), for example, lentil curry (dhal) with rice, beans with bread/tortilla. This will result in a good range of EAA being available within the body. It is not difficult but does need more planning than when a food is a complete protein.
    Antinutritional factors found in plant-based proteins can reduce the digestibility and/or availability of protein in a variety of ways such as inhibiting digestive enzymes, although food preparation techniques can mitigate some of the effects (Lynch et al., 2018). Research with 60 athletes comparing omnivore and vegetarian/vegan protein intake and protein quality concluded that vegetarians/vegans should have an additional 10 g protein per day on top of estimated requirements if aiming for 1.2 g protein/kg/day, and an additional 22 g protein per day if aiming for 1.4 g protein/kg/day. No guidance was given above this level (Ciuris et al., 2019). The lack of data in this study may have resulted in the vegetarian protein score being slightly underestimated. As practical examples, using soy milk, and using soy products such soy yoghurt, tofu and tempeh regularly, also pea protein, Quorn and quinoa in several meals per week, will ensure your protein quality is closer to that of omnivores. Check you are using mixed sources of protein and that the portion sizes are large enough (see Table 5.2 below).
2   Are you trying to build strength?
    When trying to increase strength usually resistance exercise is undertaken. This resistance exercise will result in strength gain if the load is high enough and adequate protein amounts are taken as seen above.
3   Are you recovering from an injury?
    The advice from Tipton et al. (2015) is that after injury high-protein intakes of around 2.0–2.5 g protein/kg/day can help prevent muscle loss and support recovery. Achieving an adequate protein intake after injury can be more difficult if appetite is also reduced which can happen in the face of experiencing pain and being less or differently active to

Table 5.2 Example of protein distribution across a dance day

Protein distribution across the day		
Time/meal	*Amount of protein for 55/70 kg dancer (g)*	*Example of foods*
Breakfast	20/25	Bowl of porridge made with 300 ml milk/soy milk + 1 tsp chopped nuts/nut butter and fruit/dried fruit. Add a slice of toast with nut butter for higher requirements
Midmorning snack	5/5	Bar with nuts/seeds in OR Fruit with 20 g nuts OR Breadsticks and carrots with houmous
Lunch	20/30	Sandwich with protein filling, have three to four slices bread to meet higher requirements
Midafternoon snack	5/10	Latte/cappuccino/yoghurt, dairy or soy add bar for higher requirements
Dinner	25/30	Chicken breast or 100 g firm tofu stir fry with rice and vegetables. Add lentils or chickpeas to meet the higher requirement
Dessert/evening snack	13/12	Banana loaf and mug of hot chocolate OR Greek (soy) yoghurt with added fruit and nuts plus granola as liked

your usual schedule. If immobilised it is possible that increasing EAA and/or leucine may be useful to prevent muscle loss, but more research is needed. What is known is that reducing energy intake drastically is neither necessary nor helpful: recovery needs both protein and energy. If you are experiencing an injury which will impact on activity levels significantly for a number of weeks or more, then individualised advice from an experienced qualified nutrition professional such as a dietitian is advised.

4 Are you meeting your energy needs?

As you saw in Chapter 3, carbohydrates and fats are the energy sources used for dance under normal circumstances. If you are not

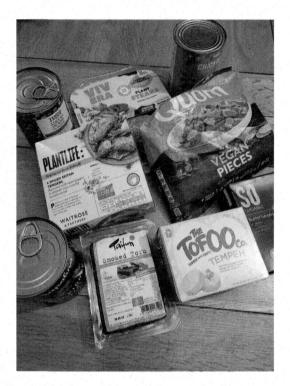

Photo 5.3 Vegan protein.

meeting your energy requirements, then there is potential for protein to be used as an energy source rather than for all of the repair and growth processes. The best solution to this situation is to increase your intake of carbohydrates and fats to meet your energy needs, rather than to try and rely on a very high intake of protein. If this is challenging then it would be useful to get individualised advice from a qualified dietitian or registered sports nutritionist who is experienced in working with dancers. If protein is substituted for necessary carbohydrate/fat you may find you are less hungry overall, which can make consuming adequate carbs and fats more difficult. This is likely to have implications for health and well-being – see Chapters 4 and 6 for more information.

5   Any other condition which may impact on your protein goals?
      If you are pregnant, have recently had surgery or have a medical condition such as Crohn's disease that may impact on protein goals, then you may well benefit from individual advice.

IV Matching intake to dance schedule

Protein and appetite

Protein is a major contributor to appetite regulation: a low-protein intake is less likely to keep you full than a diet with enough protein for your needs. If you find yourself eating what appears to be a good amount of food, for example, pasta with vegetables and a little cheese, or noodles with vegetables and a few nuts, but you get hungry quickly afterwards, then try adding some protein. This will help you reach not just your protein targets, but also add valuable vitamins and minerals.

Dancers frequently have incredibly busy and demanding schedules for many weeks of the year. When in training, these schedules may be consistent for a number of weeks, but periods of rehearsals and shows can be very different, requiring dietary planning. Within the sports world, there has been much debate and research as to the best timing for protein intake to allow the body to benefit and recover from training as constructively as possible.

It is important that protein is spread across the day, in amounts of around 20–30 g per meal for dancers under the age of 30 years (Witard et al., 2014) and up to 40 g per meal for dancers over the age of 30. There is unlikely to be benefit of having more than 40 g protein in one meal: it is better to spread the protein for the day evenly over 3–5 meals/snacks rather than focus a large proportion of the day's protein in one meal. For example, if 80% of the day's total protein is eaten in one meal, not all of it can be used for growth and repair. As protein is both expensive and scarce compared with many sources of carbohydrate and fat it is wise to divide the daily protein intake up as evenly as possible – typically breakfast will be a smaller amount than the midday or evening meals. An increase in MPS (and therefore enhanced recovery and increased strength) requires you to be in what is known as positive protein balance: you are losing less protein than you are gaining. Providing your body with an amount of protein that is enough to result in MPS every three to five hours is the strategy likely to be most effective in achieving this.

Including some protein straight after intense training – in particular resistance training – may help promote muscle adaptation. There has been much discussion between experts, as results of research have been varied due to different participant characteristics, for example, untrained or athletes. But a recent review paper has concluded that 'Regardless of training status, the acute response of muscle protein synthesis (MPS) is indicative of protein turnover and muscle remodeling critical for recovery from exercise and adaptation to training' (Witard 2021).

There are two additional reasons why it is best to spread your protein intake over three meals and one to three snacks in order to work in combination with your carb intake:

1 Protein is satiating: this means it contributes to fullness (Halton & Hu 2004). While supplements can be used – see Chapter 8 for more information on this – using food sources of protein is recommended as much as possible to optimise your nutrient intake. To eat a significant proportion of a day's protein in one meal is challenging. Meals with little protein in may leave you feeling hungry again more quickly than expected.

2 Protein-rich foods also contribute a range of other nutrients, typically micronutrients such as iron, zinc, B vitamins. Eating different protein-rich foods will provide greater variety of micronutrients which will help you reach your requirements.

Table 5.2 gives an example of how two dancers, one weighing approximately 55 kg and one weighing approximately 70 kg might distribute their protein over a day with training during the day and only a short lunch break and a free evening. The 55-kg dancer is aiming for around 88 g protein, and the 70-kg dancer is aiming for around 112 g protein.

V Practical advice and resources

Menu planning

Meeting your protein needs in an enjoyable way takes organisation, particularly if money is limited. Many dancers find it helpful to plan meals as this allows more variety to be included, can help minimise food waste and can help budgeting. This doesn't mean you can't make the most of bargains – some flexibility is always useful when translating nutrition theory into practical application. Knowing when supermarkets discount items which have a 'use-by' date approaching is useful as you may be able to get protein more cheaply to cook on the day and eat or freeze according to plans.

Food safety

i Use-by dates
  Remember that use-by dates are there to reduce the risk of food poisoning, while 'best-before dates' indicate the time when the food will taste at its best. It is unlikely any food eaten after a 'best-before' date will cause you any harm, whereas eating food after a 'use-by' date is taking a risk. US information differs from the UK, Europe and Australia at the time of writing. Australia states that food should not be consumed after a 'use-by' date as there is risk of harm, and both the UK and Europe clearly state food can cause harm after the use-by date even if it neither appears nor smells bad or different. The US currently

advises consumers to use their sense of smell. Generally, it is best to go by national guidelines, but you are best to use extreme caution with protein-rich foods because bacteria which can cause harm grow well on high-protein foods.

ii Sell-by dates and food storage

A 'sell-by' date is a guide to a store rather than a consumer in the US. When considering food safety, the over-riding principle should be to store foods according to guidelines, use within advised dates, and if a food item does not appear fresh, then don't use it. With storage comes a reduction in some vitamins so using any food that has a short shelf life soon after purchase optimises intake.

Sources of protein

For information on portion sizes providing useful amounts of protein, you are directed to Table 5.3.

Table 5.3 Portions of protein to supply 18–20 g protein

Protein portion to supply 18–20 g protein

Food	Portion size	Handy measure
Chicken breast/thigh without bone	Small breast/average thigh	Size of pack of cards
White fish	Fillet about 100 g uncooked	Size of pack of cards
Salmon fillet (no skin)	90 g raw weight	Small fillet
Eggs	Three medium whole eggs	n/a
Cheese, e.g., cheddar	60 g cheddar provides 15 g protein (6 cm × 4 cm × 2.5 cm)	½ cup grated/size of two small matchboxes
Beans, e.g., kidney beans, chick peas	1 × 400 g can be drained	Eight heaped tablespoons
Red Lentils, cooked	240 g	Seven heaped tablespoons/two heaped large serving spoons
Tofu – firm set (check labels of other types)	100 g	3/4 size of pack of cards
Quorn vegan pieces	120 g uncooked weight	24 pieces, about 1/3 dinner plate
Beef mince, lean, raw weight	100 g	Size of 1/4 lb burger
Pork or lamb steak	1 small steak	Size of pack of cards

Meat

Meat is a great source of iron and B12, and we would suggest that including red meat once or twice per week is a useful contribution to a range of nutrients. Offal – liver, kidney, and heart – while some dancers even if meat eaters may not wish to include these products, they are usually cheap and a good source of both protein and a range of micronutrients. Lean red meat is low in fat – avoid the fattier cuts of red meat, fat takes longer to digest and is less helpful in a performance diet. Trim off fat before or after cooking. Trimming before means you can control the fat content more easily, but you may get a better result if some fat is left on for cooking and then trimmed before eating. Meat that takes longer to cook, in a casserole or stew, will be cheapest. Planning for this, either to use a recipe that takes several hours to cook on the hob or in the oven, or using a slow cooker or a pressure cooker can all help achieve meals with great quality protein at less cost than using the most expensive cuts which usually cook much more quickly.

Poultry – chicken/turkey/duck/goose

Chicken and turkey meat are both high in protein low fat and typically cheaper than red meat. The leg – dark – meat with have more iron than breast meat as well as usually being more economical. Duck and goose have slightly higher fat but are still great sources of protein, as well as some micronutrients.

Game

Game, which includes venison, wild boar, hare as well as game birds such as pheasant and grouse, is high in protein and low in fat, as well as being a source of micronutrients. Often more expensive but will depend on local availability.

Fish

Fish are divided into oily fish and white fish, with seafood being a further category. All fish are an excellent source of protein. While white fish can generally be included several times per week, there are some exceptions which are looked at in this section. Oily fish need to be limited – see below. The sustainability of fish and seafood is a concern area that is explored in Chapter 12.

Sea bream, sea bass, turbot, halibut and rock salmon (also known as dogfish, flake, huss, rigg or rock eel) should not be eaten frequently:

two portions from this group per week are likely the balance between benefits and possible disadvantages. In addition, shark, marlin and swordfish can contain mercury. Eat no more than one portion of these per week, and if you are pregnant or trying to become pregnant, then avoid completely.

Oily fish

Oily fish are an excellent source of protein, as well as a number of vitamins and minerals, and omega-3 fatty acids. Oily fish include salmon, tuna, mackerel, pilchards, sardines, herring, sprats and trout. From a sustainability point of view, choosing herring, rainbow trout, anchovy and mackerel is good option – check up-to-date information on marine conservation websites. Canned fish is usually an excellent option for those with a tight budget.

There are recommendations of maximum amounts of oily fish to have weekly (on average, as this is a long-term calculation) due to the amounts of some chemicals they contain from the environment: but consensus is oily fish are still very beneficial in moderate amounts. Pre-menopausal females are advised to have no more than two portions per week. Males and older females can have up to four portions per week.

White fish

These include cod, plaice, haddock, coley, flounder, sole, sea bass, sea bream, turbot, halibut and rock salmon (dogfish/huss/rock eel). All white fish are a great source of protein and are also low in fat. Some white fish, such as sea bass and halibut, contain omega-3 fatty acids, but at lower levels than in oily fish.

Pollock and coley are more sustainable than the more well-known types of white fish.

There are no limits on the amounts of white fish that can be included weekly, but variety in sources of protein is best for meeting your overall nutritional intake.

Shellfish

Shellfish includes prawns/shrimp, mussels, scallops, squid, oysters and langoustine.

Shellfish are low in fat as well as being a source of selenium, zinc, iodine and copper.

Some types of shellfish, such as mussels, oysters, squid and crab, are also good sources of long-chain omega-3 fatty acids, but they do not contain as much as oily fish.

Shellfish are high risk when it comes to food poisoning. Take great care when buying, storing and preparing shellfish – if you are not confident then check out best practice before you shop.

Eggs

Eggs are a source not just of excellent quality protein due to the balance of amino acids; they also provide useful amounts of a number of vitamins and minerals including vitamin B12, biotin, vitamin D, phosphorous and selenium and are economical too. Both egg white and egg yolk contain good amounts of protein – in fact egg yolk has a higher amount of protein than egg white. Egg yolk contains some cholesterol, but unless you have a medical condition, such as hereditary high blood fat levels, this is not a problem and you can include eggs in several meals per week – there is no upper limit, but as always its best to include a range of foods over a week as far as is possible.

Cheese

Cheese made from the milk of animals including cows, goat sheep and buffalo can be made in a variety of ways which impact on the nutritional content. Cows' milk cheeses range from stilton, a full-fat cheese, high in salt as well as protein to cottage cheese, which is a low-fat option with a much higher water content. For those who are lactose intolerant, it may be useful to remember that most hard cheeses are carbohydrate free, so contain no lactose. Further information on food intolerances is covered in Chapter 13.

Milk

Milk, whole, semi-skimmed or skimmed, is an excellent source of the EEA leucine: if you avoid cow's milk then be sure to pick the best alternative nutritionally that you can. Sheep and goat's milk are comparable with cow's milk for total protein, though lower in leucine. Currently, soy has the next highest amount of total protein, at over 3 g per 100 ml, followed by some pea milk substitutes and oat milk substitutes which provide over 2 g protein per 100 ml. Check before you buy: many of the nut-based alternatives to milk contain very little protein as the nut content is very low. Cow's milk is over 3 g protein per 100 ml, dairy alternatives can be as low as 0.1 g protein per 100 ml, which if you have milk in porridge/on cereal and in drinks over the day could easily result in a protein difference of 10 g per day, which is significant.

Soy/tempeh/tofu

Soy protein is hugely useful in many areas of the world, and is available in a number of formats which can easily be included in meals. It is a high-quality protein and including it in several meals per week will support maintaining good quality protein intake. It can also contribute useful amounts of iron to your diet.

Quorn

Quorn products are widely available in many countries. Quorn is made from mycoprotein – a protein that is similar to that found in mushroom, and only the concentration is much higher in Quorn. While the protein content is excellent, it is not a great source of iron, so you would benefit from including beans, lentils, dark green leafy veg and/or peas in a meal with Quorn.

Seitan

Seitan is in fact gluten, derived from wheat. It is not a complete protein so be sure to include a range of other (non-grain) proteins over the day.

Newer products such pea protein products and 'vegan meat substitutes'

The range is growing, and many new products may be both great tasting and have a good protein content. See Chapter 12 for more on this topic.

It's worth checking labels – there are products labelled as 'vegan meat substitute' that have minimal protein, such as banana blossom and jackfruit. Many vegan cheese substitutes are just oil and starch with negligible protein. If you wish to use products for flavour rather than nutrition that is of course fine, but check you are getting what you expected when buying alternatives to conventional foods. Table 5.3 shows portions of protein-rich foods that will each supply 18–20 g protein.

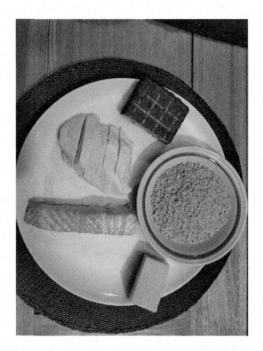

Photo 5.4 Examples of protein portion sizes for tofu, salmon, chicken, lentils and cheese

VI Resources

The vegan athlete's cookbook: Author Anita Bean 2021, published by Bloomsbury.

Plant Power: Annie Bell 2020, published by Kyle Books.

Joanisse, S., McKendry, J., Lim, C., Nunes, E.A., Stokes, T., Mcleod, J.C., and Phillips, SM. (2021). Understanding the effects of nutrition and post-exercise nutrition on skeletal muscle protein turnover: Insights from stable isotope studies. *Clinical Nutrition Open Science*, 36, pp. 56–77.

Gilani, G.S., Cockell, K.A., Sepehr, E. (2005). Effects of antinutritional factors on protein digestibility and amino acid availability in foods. *Journal of AOAC International*, 88(3), pp. 967–987.

Snijders, T., Trommelen, J., Kouw, I.W., Holwerda, A.M., Verdijk, L.B., Van Loon, L.J. (2019). The impact of pre-sleep protein ingestion on the skeletal muscle adaptive response to exercise in humans: an update. *Frontiers in Nutrition*, 17.

VII Learning outcomes

After reading this chapter the reader should be able to:

1 Explain the difference between essential and non-EEA.
2 Discuss why dancers need more protein than sedentary individuals.
3 State nutritional differences between vegetarian and animal sources of protein.
4 Explain why and how protein should be distributed over the day's meals and snacks.

References

Biolo, G. et al. (1995) Increased rates of muscle protein turnover and amino acid transport after resistance exercise in humans, *American Journal of Physiology-Endocrinology and Metabolism*, 268(3), pp.E514–E520.

Brown, M.A., Stevenson, E.J. and Howatson, G. (2018) Whey protein hydrolysate supplementation accelerates recovery from exercise-induced muscle damage in females, *Applied Physiology, Nutrition, and Metabolism,* 43(4), pp.324–330.

Ciuris, C. et al. (2019) A comparison of dietary protein digestibility, based on DIAAS scoring, in vegetarian and non-vegetarian athletes, *Nutrients,* 11(12), pp.3016.

Deen, D. et al. (2021) Identification of the transcription factor MAZ as a regulator of erythropoiesis, *Blood Advances*, 5(15), pp.3002–3015.

Devries, M.C. et al. (2018) Leucine, not total protein, content of a supplement is the primary determinant of muscle protein anabolic responses in healthy older women, *The Journal of Nutrition*, 148(7), pp.1088–1095.

Gorissen, S.H. et al. (2018) Protein content and amino acid composition of commercially available plant-based protein isolates, *Amino Acids,* 50(12), pp.1685–1695.

Halton, T.L. and Hu, F.B. (2004) The effects of high protein diets on thermogenesis, satiety and weight loss: A critical review, *Journal of the American College of Nutrition,* 23(5), pp.373–385.

Hodson, N. et al. (2019) Molecular regulation of human skeletal muscle protein synthesis in response to exercise and nutrients: A compass for overcoming age-related anabolic resistance, *American Journal of Physiology-Cell Physiology*, 317(-6), pp.C1061–C1078.

Jackman, S.R. et al. (2017) Branched-chain amino acid ingestion stimulates muscle myofibrillar protein synthesis following resistance exercise in humans, *Frontiers in Physiology*, 8, pp.390.

Lynch, H., Johnston, C. and Wharton, C. (2018) Plant-based diets: Considerations for environmental impact, protein quality, and exercise performance, *Nutrients,* 10(12), pp.1841.

Morton, R.W., Colenso-Semple, L. and Phillips, S.M. (2019) Training for strength and hypertrophy: An evidence-based approach, *Current Opinion in Physiology,* 10, pp.90–95.

Newsholme, E.A. and Blomstrand, E. (2006) Branched-chain amino acids and central fatigue, *The Journal of Nutrition*, 136(1), pp.274S–276S.

Norton, L.E. et al. (2012) Leucine content of dietary proteins is a determinant of postprandial skeletal muscle protein synthesis in adult rats, *Nutrition & Metabolism,* 9(1), pp.1–9.

Rahmanto, A.S. and Davies, M.J. (2012) Selenium-containing amino acids as direct and indirect antioxidants, *IUBMB Life*, 64(11), pp.863–871.

Reggiani, C. and Schiaffino, S. (2020) Muscle hypertrophy and muscle strength: Dependent or independent variables? A provocative review, *European Journal of Translational Myology*, 30(3), pp. 9311–9323.

Shiraki, K., Yamada, T. and Yoshimura, H. (1977) Relation of protein nutrition to the reduction of red blood cells induced by physical training, *The Japanese Journal of Physiology*, 27(4), pp.413–421.

Thomas, D.T., Erdman, K.A., Burke, L.M. (2016) Position of the Academy of Nutrition and Dietetics, Dietitians of Canada, and the American College of Sports Medicine: Nutrition and athletic performance. *Journal of the Academy of Nutrition and Dietetics*, 116(3), pp.501–528.

Tipton, K.D. (2015) Nutritional support for exercise-induced injuries, *Sports Medicine*, 45(1), pp.93–104.

Volpi, E., Nazemi, R. and Fujita, S. (2004) Muscle tissue changes with aging, *Current Opinion in Clinical Nutrition and Metabolic Care*, 7(4), pp.405.

Witard, O.C., Bannock, L. and Tipton, K.D. (2021) Making sense of muscle protein synthesis: A focus on muscle growth during resistance training, *International Journal of Sport Nutrition and Exercise Metabolism*, 1(aop), pp.1–13.

Witard, O.C., Garthe, I. and Phillips, S.M. (2019) Dietary protein for training adaptation and body composition manipulation in track and field athletes, *International Journal of Sport Nutrition and Exercise Metabolism*, 29(2), pp.165–174.

Witard, O.C. et al. (2014) Myofibrillar muscle protein synthesis rates subsequent to a meal in response to increasing doses of whey protein at rest and after resistance exercise, *The American Journal of Clinical Nutrition*, 99(1), pp.86–95.

Witard, O.C. et al. (2016) Growing older with health and vitality: A nexus of physical activity, exercise and nutrition, *Biogerontology*, 17(3), pp.529–546.

Zaromskyte, G. et al. (2021) Evaluating the leucine trigger hypothesis to explain the postprandial regulation of muscle protein synthesis in young and older adults: A systematic review, *Frontiers in Nutrition*, 8, pp.402.

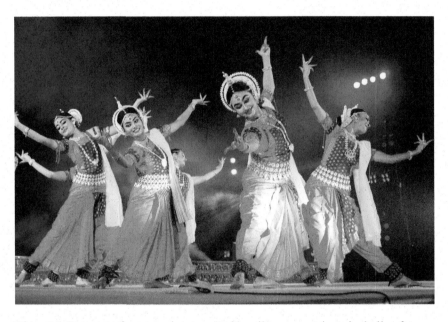

Photo 6.1 Dance performance is supported by all macronutrients including fats.
Credit: ShaikhMeraj/Shutterstock

6 Dietary fat for health and longevity

Contents

Fats myth	Fats truth
Fat is unnecessary/fat makes you fat	Fat is a necessary fuel for the body and is also needed structurally, i.e. to protect your organs. It is also key for hormone production and function, but fat won't be stored if you are meeting your energy needs.
All saturated fat is bad	Saturated fat is found naturally in many foods. Meeting fat requirements, and focussing on plant-based oils in cooking will help you have a suitable balance of fats in your meals for both health and performance.
Cholesterol is bad for you	Cholesterol is needed to make vitamin D and some hormones. High blood cholesterol is often due to genetics: most people don't need a low cholesterol diet.
A high-fat diet is best for endurance performance	Fat is slow to digest. Even though some dance is low intensity, dance almost always involves high-intensity activity, fuelled by carbs, and a high fat diet will limit carb intake. Having around 1/3 of your energy intake from fat will work well.

(Continued)

DOI: 10.4324/9781003219002-6

Table 6.1 (Continued)

Fats myth	Fats truth
All fat free foods are good for you	Foods that naturally have very little fat, such as fruit and veg, are an important part of the dancer's diet. Foods that are manufactured to be low fat/fat free often have been highly processed, and sugar may be used to add more flavour. Choose less processed foods to make up the main part of your diet.

I Introduction

'Lipids' is the chemical term for fats and oils, though in humans, 'lipids' tends to be used when talking about the levels of different types of fats in the blood, while 'fats' is the term most often used when referring to food.

There are many different chemical structures within the fats and oils 'family', all composed of just three different chemical elements – carbon, hydrogen and oxygen. These differences result in different properties and uses in cooking. The difference between fats and carbohydrates – which also contain only carbon, hydrogen and oxygen – is the ratios of these elements to one another. This difference results in different energy content as well as different rates of digestion, and speed of use by our bodies. Fats have many roles, not just providing crucial energy to the body, but also supporting cell growth and allowing fat-soluble vitamins to be digested and to reach target cells in the body. In addition, a normal fat intake supports the immune system and has a role in controlling blood pressure.

Lipids/fats don't readily dissolve in water – when oil is mixed with water it will remain separate, although it is possible to improve the level of mixing and make an emulsion – such as when making an oil and vinegar salad dressing – by mixing vigorously. This emulsion is unstable and will separate out over time, so to keep water and oil mixed together there needs to be an emulsifier – for example mayonnaise doesn't separate into the water/vinegar and oil components due to the presence of lecithin, a natural emulsifier found in egg yolks (and other foods, including soya beans). This separation is important when thinking about nutrients that are found mostly in high-fat foods, such as vitamin E: a diet low in fat will be low in vitamin E too. For more on vitamin E, see Appendix A.

Lipids are required for every physiological process in the body. As they are energy dense, with over twice the energy content of carbohydrate and protein, and not bulky, it is easier to eat enough compared with protein and carb, but dancers still benefit from paying attention to the amounts and choices of fats in the diet as this can impact on performance.

As there are different types of fats with different effects within the body, there can be confusing advice surrounding fats. It can be useful to remember that thinking about fat as a fuel is a short-term focus, whereas concern about the types of fats in the diet is a longer-term health focus.

Over recent decades, there have been swings in how carbohydrates and fats have been seen, particularly in the media, and there have been many trends often labelling either fats or carbs as 'bad'. There is a real problem here, as the media wants a story that is very black or white: that individual foods are 'good' or 'bad'. But in nutrition, unless a food is going to cause harm – for example, because it hasn't been stored properly and has spoilt – no food can be labelled 100% 'bad' or 'unhealthy'. It is important to remember it's the amount and frequency of foods that you eat which makes your overall diet more or less healthy.

Fats have the highest energy density (9 kcal per g of fat) out of the energy-providing macronutrients. This is useful when looking for low-volume foods to provide a high amount of energy. For performers, nuts and seeds are examples of useful high-fat/energy-dense foods: mixed with some dried fruit, or as nut or seed butter with fruit/crackers, they can provide a snack which is less bulky than a carb only snack, often more palatable, and with a bigger range of nutrients: the downside is the slower digestion and metabolism of fats (which will be looked at shortly) to help you achieve a ratio of fats to carbs that will best support dance and performance.

II Different types of fats and their relevance to health and performance

Understanding some of the science behind the different types of fat can help you make the most appropriate choices when thinking about your own food intake. Figure 6.1 shows the different types of fats required by dancers.

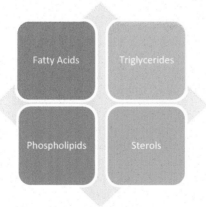

Figure 6.1 Types of fats needed by dancers.

i **Fatty acids**

These are the simplest of fats. Their structure is a long chain of carbons bonded together, with a carboxyl group (one atom of carbon is joined to two of oxygen, and one of the oxygen molecules is also joined to a hydrogen atom) at one end.

Fatty acids are described as short, medium and long:

- Short-chain fatty acids (less than eight units), which tend to be liquid at room temperature.
- Medium-chain fatty acids (8–12). These are also usually liquid at room temperature.
- Long-chain fatty acids (>12): more likely to be solid at room temperature, especially if they are saturated:
- Links or bonds between carbon–carbon bonds can either be single or double.
- In saturated fatty acids, all carbon-carbon bonds are single bonds (Figure 6.2).

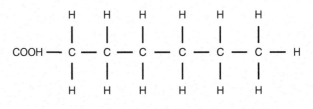

SATURATED FAT

Figure 6.2 The generic structure of saturated fatty acid.

Examples of saturated fats are:

Lauric acid (12 carbon) found in coconut oil and palm oil.
Myristic acid (14 carbons) found in cow's milk and dairy products.
Palmitic acid (16 carbons) found in palm oil, lard and meat.
Stearic acid (18 carbons) found in meat.

Practical note:
A high intake of saturated fats is widely accepted as the main cause of raised cholesterol levels, so there are recommendations on upper limits of around 10% of your energy intake. This is unlikely to be a problem for any dancer following guidelines given later in the chapter.

In unsaturated fatty acids, there are one or more double bonds (i.e., not all bonds are saturated with hydrogen). From a food perspective, this means that unsaturated fatty acids melt at cooler temperatures compared to saturated fats of the same chain length. The more unsaturated bonds a fatty acid has, the more likely it is to be liquid at room temperature. Unsaturated fatty acids need to make up the majority of a dancer's fat intake.

Monounsaturated fatty acids have one double bond. In the illustration, the double bond is indicated by the bold arrow in Figure 6.3.

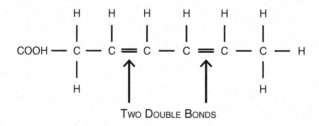

MONOUNSATURATED FAT

Figure 6.3 The generic structure of a monounsaturated fatty acid.

Monounsaturated fatty acids (sometimes abbreviated as MUFA) are found mainly in plants (oils, avocado, nuts and seeds).

Examples include:

Oleic fatty acids (found in olive oil, sesame, peanut): 18 carbons in a chain, has one double bond, which is at the ninth carbon in the chain from the methyl (CH3 group, written 18:1 w-9.

Erucic fatty acids (rapeseed oil) 22:1 w-9.

The 'w' denotes where on the carbon chain the first double bond appears.

Polyunsaturated fatty acids (PUFAs) have more than one double bond. In Figure 6.4, the double bonds are indicated by the bold arrows.

```
          H    H    H    H    H    H
          |    |    |    |    |    |
COOH  —   C  — C  = C  — C  = C  — C  —  H
          |         ↑         ↑         |
          H         |         |         H
                TWO DOUBLE BONDS
```

POLYUNSATURATED FAT

Figure 6.4 The generic structure of a polyunsaturated fatty acid.

Categories of PUFAs

PUFAs are categorised according to the location of the first double bond in the carbon chain.

If the first double bond is between the third and fourth carbon (from the methyl CH$_3$), the fatty acids are known as omega-3 (w-3). This group includes

- Alpha-linolenic acid (ALA) which contains 18 carbon atoms and can be found in some types of vegetable oil.
- Eicosapentaenoic (EPA) which contains 20 carbons found in fish oil.
- Docosahexaenoic (DHA) which contains 22 carbons also found in fish oil.

These are the most well-known and understood omega-3 fats.

As the human body can't synthesise the double bonds in omega-3 (and omega-6 which will be explored shortly), the omega-3 fatty acid ALA is an essential fatty acid (EFA): therefore, you need to get it from food or supplements.

Although ALA can be converted into EPA and then to DHA, the proportion converted (which occurs mainly in the liver) is very limited and possibly less in young men (Burdge et al., 2002) than in young women (Burdge & Wooton, 2002).

Consuming EPA and DHA directly from foods and/or dietary supplements is the only practical way to increase levels of these fatty acids in the body, and EPA and DHA are usually referred to as EFAs.

If the first double bond is between carbon 6–7 (counting from the methyl CH3), the fatty acids are known as omega-6 (w-6). This group includes

- Linoleic fatty acid which is found in vegetable oils – see below.

Linoleic acid is an EFA. Unlike the omega-3 fatty acids, linoleic acid is abundant in many vegetable oils, and the risk of deficiency is low unless total fat intake is well below recommended levels.

There are additional classifications for fatty acids, based on the position of hydrogen molecules on the carbons at the double bond.

In cis fatty acids which are most naturally occurring fatty acids, both hydrogen atoms are on same side. The cis bond causes the carbon 'backbone' of the fatty acid to bend as shown in Figure 6.5

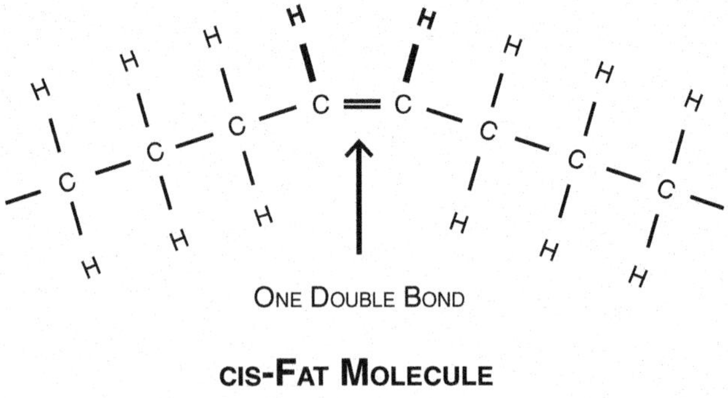

ONE DOUBLE BOND

cis-Fat Molecule

Figure 6.5 The generic structure of cis fatty acids.

Trans fats are almost exclusively found after oils have been processed, by the addition of an extra hydrogen atom, for example to make some margarines and foods containing margarines, such as cakes and biscuits. In trans fats, the hydrogen atoms are on opposite sides of the carbon 'backbone' of the fatty acid. Fatty acids with a trans bond remain straight, similar to saturated fat, and are more likely, therefore, to be solid at room temperature. They are unsaturated fats (Figure 6.6).

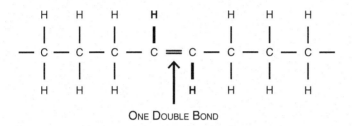

ONE DOUBLE BOND

TRANS-FAT MOLECULE

Figure 6.6 The generic structure of trans fatty acids.

ii Triglycerides (TAG)

Triglyceride is the commonly used name for triacylglycerols, hence the abbreviation TAG. Structurally TAG's are three fatty acids (saturated/unsaturated or both) attached to a glycerol (form of glucose) molecule, as shown in Figure 6.7. TAG account for 95% of dietary fat.

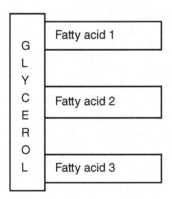

Figure 6.7 The generic structure of triglycerides.

The digestion of triglycerides

While carbohydrates and proteins are soluble in water, TAG are not. In addition they are large molecules. In the gut, TAG cluster in large droplets;

this makes digestion more challenging. Lipases are the enzymes which are responsible for the digestion of fats. While some lipase is produced in the tongue, this seems to only have a small role in adults though it is useful for babies (Hamosh, 1990). Lipase is also produced in the stomach, and the pancreas from where it is released into the small intestine. Overall during the whole digestion period, gastric (stomach) lipase might be responsible for under 20% of the digestion that is required (Carriere et al., 1993). From a practical point of view, the majority of TAGs are digested in the small intestine. The chyme – partially digested food – moving from the stomach to the small intestine contains lipids which are clustered in large droplets.

Bile, which is produced by the liver and usually stored in the gall bladder before it is released into the first part of the small intestine, acts as an emulsifier and breaks the TAGs into small droplets. TAGs can then be broken down to fatty acids, glycerol and monoglycerides by pancreatic lipase.

In the small intestine, the fatty acids and glycerol along with fat-soluble vitamins and cholesterol from food form complexes called micelles with bile salts, which helps absorption.

The contents of these micelles enter the enterocytes (epithelial cells lining the small intestine). There the bile salts separate again and are recycled. The short and medium-chain fatty acids and glycerol are absorbed directly into the bloodstream. Long-chain fatty acids and monoglycerides reassemble into TAG, and together with fat-soluble vitamins, and cholesterol, are incorporated into chylomicrons for transport. Chylomicrons, which are lipoproteins, enter the lymphatic system and from there enter the bloodstream to reach the liver and other body tissues.

Practical implications

Fat is digested slowly compared to carbohydrates. The advice to get 20–35% of energy from fat allows you to meet your daily essential requirements; the slowing effect on digestion means not being hungry too quickly, but also you are not struggling with being full for hours after very high-fat foods. Of course, 20–35% is an average; you can, and should, enjoy a range of foods with a variety of fat contents. But prior to training and performance, it is best to keep to lower fat options so your stomach isn't busy digesting food while you are tackling challenging dance moves in class, rehearsal or on stage.

iii **Phospholipids**
Phospholipids are the third category of lipids. Phospholipids are needed by the human body: they can be obtained from food but also can be made by the body.
Structure of phospholipids
Phospholipids are similar to TAG however one fatty acid is replaced by a phosphate group. Each phospholipid is made up of two fatty acids, a phosphate group, and a glycerol molecule.

Function of phospholipids

Phospholipids have many functions within a cell (Dowhan, 1997). They are the main component of our cell membranes. In addition, they provide the supporting matrix and surface for catalytic processes and are involved in signalling mechanisms to control what happens within cells.

iv **Sterols**

Sterols are the final group of compounds that are classed as fats, although as well as containing fatty acids, their structure chemically is that of an alcohol – a solid one that will not have any of the effects of ethanol (the substance usually thought of when people think of alcohol). It is the oxygen with hydrogen group that is the alcohol group chemically.

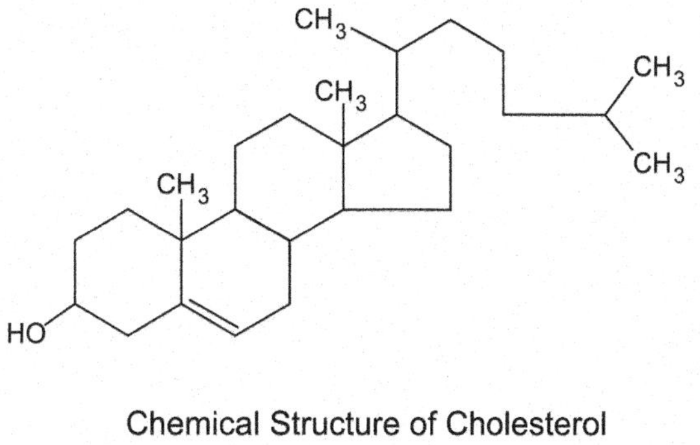

Chemical Structure of Cholesterol

Photo 6.2 Chemical structure of cholesterol.
Credit: Kicky_Princess/Shutterstock

Function of sterols

The sterol you are likely most familiar with is cholesterol. In fact, all tissues in the body can manufacture cholesterol, and 90% of cholesterol is found in your cell membranes.

Cholesterol is also part of myelin, the outer coating of nerve cells.

Although cholesterol tends to have a bad reputation, this is far from the full picture. There are different types of cholesterol which have different impacts on health. In addition, cholesterol is essential for health: it is adapted within the body to synthesise steroid hormones, bile acid and vitamin D – this last one also requires the presence of sunlight – see Appendix A.

Ergosterol, another example of a sterol, is a precursor of vitamin D found in mushrooms, which can be activated when mushrooms are exposed to adequate sunlight.

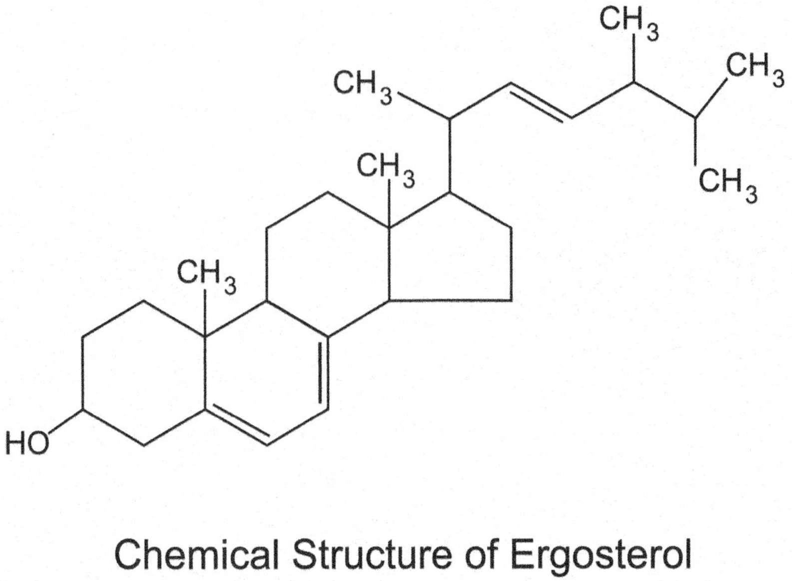

Chemical Structure of Ergosterol

Photo 6.3 Chemical structure of ergosterol.
Credit: Kicky_Princess/Shutterstock

Plant sterols have a role in reducing raised cholesterol levels. There are specialised food products where sterols have been added for this purpose.

A brief note on the transport of lipids round the body

As with the digestion of fats, the process of absorbing fats into the body and transporting them to the cells that need them is more complex than for protein and carbs, and takes longer. As discussed in the section on digestion of fats, lipoproteins help transport cholesterol, lipids and fat-soluble vitamins from the small intestine and also liver. There are three main types:

• High-density lipoproteins (HDL)
• Low-density lipoproteins (LDL)
• Chylomicrons

While HDL can remove excess cholesterol from tissues and the blood, LDL can deposit cholesterol in arteries and other body tissues.

There are ratios of HDL: LDL which are recognised as more or beneficial. Unless you have a family history of abnormal cholesterol levels, it is likely your levels and ratios will be in the normal range. Low weight and low energy intake can cause abnormally high levels temporarily, which will resolve when nutrition and health improve.

The role of the liver in fat metabolism

Your liver is simultaneously responsible for many roles in digestion. Those linked to fat digestion and metabolism are useful to consider here.

To start with though, it is useful to remember that nutrients do not exist in isolation. The body is able to do some interconversions of macronutrients – though carbs and fats can never be turned into protein, and it is not possible to convert fats directly to carbs.

In the liver, depending on factors such as glycogen stores excess protein, carbohydrate and alcohol can be converted to TAG or cholesterol. TAG made in the liver are incorporated into lipoproteins which can transport lipids out of the liver to body cells for use. Cholesterol can be transported to the liver or any organs needing it.

If you would like to look at this system in more detail a link is given in the resources section.

Sources of fat in the diet

What is in a typical oil?

Pouring out a spoonful of oil to use in a stir fry, or on a salad, you will be looking at a collection of different compounds which all contribute to the unique character of the oil.

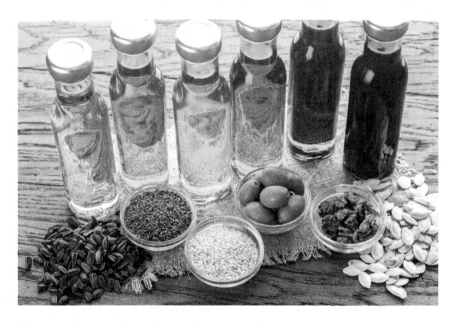

Photo 6.4 Sources of plant based oils.
Credit: Alexander Prokopenko/Shutterstock

Olive oil, for example, is about 99% TAGs (~99%) with a small amount of free fatty acids, and a mixture of other lipids such as sterols, tocopherols, and pigments, together with compounds which provide flavour.

High- and low-fat foods

A useful way of looking at sources of fat in the diet is whether they are derived from animal sources or plant sources. Almost every food contains some fat, but the amount can range from a trace amount – less than a gram – in a serving of that food and up to foods which are almost exclusively fats. Whilst it is true to say that there are a large number of plant foods which naturally have a very low-fat content, there are also foods of animal origin that have a very low-fat content, for example, some types of white fish, egg whites, skimmed milk and very low-fat yogurts, white meats (chicken and turkey), game and cottage cheese.

Significant animal sources of fat in the human diet include meat fat, butter and most cheeses. Eggs and oily fish are moderate sources of fat.

Types of food oils and their benefits

Type of oil	Uses in cooking	Nutritional benefits
Olive oil	Extra virgin olive oil : salad dressing Olive oil: roasting, shallow fry Can be used in standard cooking temperatures (120–200°C)	High in antioxidants and rich in flavour
Rapeseed/Canola oil	Very good choice for baking, roasting and salad dressings	Good balance of fatty acids Good source of ALA fats (omega-3 fats) Rich source of Vit K
Sunflower seed oil	Good choice for any use, it can be used at high temperatures	Low in saturates, source of Vit E and Vit K
Peanut oil	Stir fry	Good source of monounsaturated fats
Sesame seed oil	Salad dressing, stir fry	Low in saturated fat, source of antioxidants
Hemp oil	Salad dressing, dip	Source of omega 3
Flaxseed/linseed oil (should not be exposed to heat)	Salad dressing, dip	Good source of omega 3
Soybean oil	Stir fry	Vit K, Vit E, can lower cholesterol
Walnut oil (should not be exposed to heat)	Salad dressing, add to cooked veg/pasta	Some omega 3, Vit K, low in saturates

Significant plant sources of fat are vegetable oils and spreads, seeds and nuts and avocados.

Meat and dairy fat have a higher proportion of saturated fat than most plant sources, coconut oil is one exception. Manufactured snack foods can also have a high proportion of saturated fats due to the type of fats used and sometimes due to manufacturing processes. Opting for lean meat most of the time, keeping cream for occasional use, not relying only on cheese for protein and limiting manufactured foods such as cakes and biscuits will keep saturated fat intake down, which is the recommendation for long-term health. Using plant-based oils for cooking will balance the ratios as these are high in unsaturated fats.

Trans fats

Trans fats are regarded as unhelpful for health: cis fats are the best option. The main source of trans fats is currently processed foods, where cis fats can be converted to trans fats in some manufacturing processes. Manufacturers have been working hard over the last few years to address this issue and overall levels are falling. If you are following overall dance guidelines, you are likely to be well within the recommendations for trans-fat intakes.

III Fat utilisation during dance

Measuring the proportions of fuels – carbs and fats – a dancer is using when exercising, requires equipment that is not often available. Unlike an activity where the intensity is relatively consistent, such as running on a treadmill, in dance the proportions of each type of fuel used will change according to how intensive activity is. Fat is used for low-intensity activities, and as exercise intensity increases the body uses progressively more carbohydrate and less fat.

Overall the proportion of energy from fat for athletes is recommended to be from 20% to 35% (Thomas et al., 2016). If fat intake is under 15% of energy intake, then not only will the diet be bulky, it may well be low in EFAs – these are specific fats which you need from foods, you cannot adapt other fats to make these. There is no benefit, and some risk, to reducing the amount of energy from fat below 20% (Thomas, 2016).

Looking at percentages of energy from fat isn't practical when it comes to thinking about food choices. The good news for those who find amounts useful is that the energy percentages can be converted into around one gram of fat per kg body weight. For a demanding day, as well as increasing your carb intake – see Chapter 4 – your fat intake can also be increased. As fat provides more energy gram for gram than carbohydrate, an increase to 1.25–1.5 g fat per kg body weight will meet the needs of many dancers. Dancers with high energy requirements may find that around 2 g fat per kg body weight is needed, as well as up to 7–10 g carb per kg body weight.

Practical ways to meet your needs for fats: how dancers can get the right amounts of fats:

1   Use modest amounts of suitable oil in cooking (1–2 tbsp.) such as olive oil or rapeseed oil: 1–2 tbsp oil per portion works well in many recipes, for example, rapeseed oil in a stir fry, olive oil to roast veggies.
2   Include fats from fruits, nuts and seeds in meals/snacks.
         For example, put some avocado or nut butter on toast as an alternative to spread, or use avocado or nuts/seeds on salad.
3   Choose lower-fat dairy products, for example semi-skimmed milk, feta or mozzarella rather than stilton cheese or yoghurt rather than cream.
4   Include oily fish (e.g., salmon, mackerel, sardines) once or twice each week.
5   Reduce intake of higher-fat processed foods (cakes, biscuits, pastries, crisps): use scones, fruit bread, malt loaf, banana bread and crackers instead.
6   Stir fry, grill, bake, boil or steam rather than deep frying.
7   Use small amounts of oil for any frying (1–2 tbsps per person).

Table 6.1 shows an example of food to meet fat energy goals.
NB: In Table 6.1 smaller amounts of fats for those with lower requirements, higher amounts for those with higher requirements. Carb portions need to be suitable to meet energy needs, protein portions to meet protein needs.

Table 6.1 A sample day to meet fat energy goals

Meal	Food
Breakfast	Porridge made with semi-skimmed or soya milk with fruit or dried fruit ADD: Toast with 2–3 tsp nut butter per slice if wanted
Snack	Cereal bar: look for at least 3:1 ratio of grams of carb: fat
Lunch	Protein, e.g. tuna/Quorn, with salad with 1–2 tbsp dressing and carb, e.g. a portion of bread/grains with 1–2 tbsp spread/oil Fruit and popcorn
Mid-afternoon snack	Banana bread
Dinner	Stir fry with veg, chicken/tofu and rice/noodles Yoghurt/soya yoghurt and fruit
Evening snack	Bowl of cereal with milk

Optimising fat intake for performance eating plans

Less suitable choice	More suitable choice
Sausage roll	Eggs on toast
Crisps	Dried fruit and nut mix, unsalted or lightly salted popcorn
Readymade sandwich fillers based on mayonnaise	Make your own mix to optimise the protein/mayo balance, e.g. egg mayo, tuna mayo
Cakes and doughnuts	Malt loaf, fruit bread, fruit teacake, homemade energy balls
Most biscuits	Plain biscuits, crackers, oatcakes with topping, rice cakes
Pastries	Wholegrain bagels, fruit teacake, banana bread
Double cream	Whipping cream, Greek yoghurt, silken tofu
Coconut milk (such as in curries)	Replace some with Greek yoghurt, plant milk substitute
Sausages	Plant-based sausages – check protein/fat content

IV Essential fatty acids and dance performance

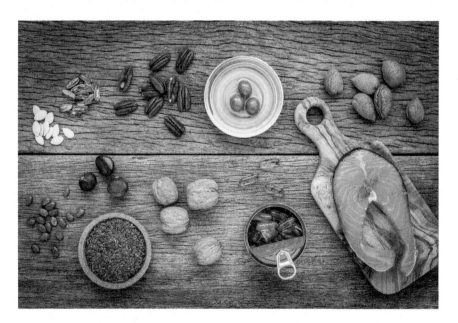

Photo 6.5 Sources of omega 3 fatty acids.
Credit: Kerdkanno/Shutterstock

In your body, EFA's are needed in particular to:

1 Make eicosanoids (made at site of tissue damage or infection):
   - There are several classes of eicosanoids: prostaglandins, thromboxanes and leukotrienes.
   - When a blood vessel is injured, thromboxane stimulates the formation of a blood clot.
   - Thromboxane also causes the muscle in the blood vessel wall to contract.
   - Prostaglandin has the opposite effect to thromboxane.
   - The opposing effects result in thromboxane and prostaglandin controlling the amount of blood flow and regulating the response to injury and inflammation.

2 Help your body recover from exercise-induced muscle damage:
   - Exercise is well known to induce damage to muscle fibres and cause inflammation.
   - EFA combat this and help to regulate the inflammatory response in the body.

Summary of the body systems impacted by EFA deficiency for the dancer

If you are vegetarian or vegan, omega-3 EFA deficiency is a risk, as the conversion from plant-based sources of ALA to EPA and DHA is low. Over the last few years, it has become more clear that EFA are involved in many areas of health and well-being. As omega-6 deficiency is only likely on a very low-fat diet, the concern is the consequences of omega-3 deficiency.

The roles of omega-3

There is increasing evidence EPA and DHA are involved in:

- Visual function
- Cognitive function
- Metabolism
- Inflammation
- Immune response
- Oxidative stress
- Wound healing
- Organ function (liver, kidney, heart, muscle)

The evidence from research is now strong enough that claims that omega-3 can help with normalising raised blood pressure, high TAG levels and heart function are permitted. Sport data are still at an early stage, with research only on small numbers of athletes. Lewis et al. (2020) have published a useful review on the topic of whether fish oil supplements offer benefits to athletes. Previous data from two research studies (Jouris et al., 2011; Corder et al., 2016) has suggested the following benefits of omega-3 in exercise. The participants weren't athletes or dancers, but the conclusions confirm the importance of EFA for these benefits:

- Optimal oxygen and nutrients to cells (blood viscosity)
- Enhanced aerobic metabolism
- Post exercise soreness minimised
- Anti-inflammatory (preventing joint, tendon, ligament strains)*
- Reduced inflammation from over-training*
- Assisted injury healing

*See Chapter 11 for discussion on the role of inflammation in exercise.

How to get enough essential fatty acids

As you saw earlier, EFAs from the omega-3 and omega-6 classes of polyunsaturated fats have to be obtained directly from food. The amount of omega-3 fats recommended is between 250 and 500 mg combined EPA and DHA each day. One to two portions of oily fish per week will cover this range.

A supplement to provide about 450 mg of EPA and DHA daily is the alternative if you don't eat oily fish.

Omega-3 from other sources – food and supplements

If your diet doesn't include oily fish, foods that have omega-3 added can be useful sources. Eggs are the most likely option, but check other foods, such as milk, and milk alternatives, or supplemented white fish products to see if there are any options that might be useful.

Although nuts and seeds, and their oils contain ALA – walnuts, flaxseeds and rapeseed oil are particularly good sources, the concern, as mentioned before, is that the conversion from ALA to EPA and DHA is low.

Algal oil is the best option for non-fish eaters as fish get their omega-3 from sea algae, so you are going direct to the fishes' source of omega-3 fatty acids.

Oily fish, omega-3 content and health notes:

Omega-3 rich foods include many types of oily fish. These are: salmon, mackerel, trout, pilchards, sardines, kippers, herring, swordfish, sprats, whitebait and fresh crab. Tuna is no longer classed as an oily fish, neither the fresh nor tinned versions. It will contain some omega-3 fatty acids but less than oily fish.

Aim for at least two portions of fish per week, of which one to two should be oily fish. Dancers who may become pregnant in the future are advised to have no more than two portions of oily fish per week on average. This is because while oily fish have many nutritional benefits, they may also contain more pollutants than other fish which may have an impact on the development of an unborn child. Omega-3 (and other) supplements containing vitamin A should also be avoided if you are pregnant or trying to become pregnant.

White fish omega-3 content and health notes

White fish, including cod, haddock, plaice, pollack, coley and Dover sole, and also shellfish contain some EPA and DHA, but at much lower levels than oily fish. On a general health note, there are some types of white fish which shouldn't be eaten too often because they contain pollutants. These include sea bass, turbot, halibut, sea bream and rock salmon – which has a number of names including dogfish, flake, huss, rigg or rock eel. Brown meat from crabs shouldn't be eaten too often for the same reason. You are advised to have no more than one portion of shark, marlin and swordfish per week as the mercury content can be high, and to avoid these altogether if you are pregnant, or are trying to get pregnant.

Omega-6

Omega-6 fats

Omega-6 fats are needed for a number of functions within the body. These include supporting normal growth and development, maintaining bone health, regulating metabolism, and maintaining the reproductive system. They also play a crucial role in brain function, and cell membranes and skin health.

Unlike omega-3 fats, most dancers are likely to eat sufficient amounts of omega-6 from spreads and vegetable oils. Providing you are including healthy amounts of fats you are likely to have an adequate intake. If you are on a very low-fat intake, then addressing this should resolve the problem of a low intake of omega-6 fatty acids.

Until there is more detailed evidence on EFA requirements for dancers ensuring you are getting adequate intakes of omega-3 whether from food, or a daily supplement would seem the best current strategy. You are encouraged to take note of ongoing research whether in dance or sport as recommendations may change over time.

V A review of high fat and ketogenic diets

There is no specific definition of a high fat diet, though it is typically recognised as a diet that provides at least 35% energy from fat. At just above 35% fat there is unlikely to be any significant effect on most dancers, unless they have a very high-intensity workload, when carbohydrate requirements will be higher than normal to fuel this fast fuel-burning workload. As fat levels increase, assuming protein stays the same – which is not a given, but is possible to achieve – then carb intakes will have to fall to maintain energy balance. This will impact on glycogen levels, which will impact on your ability to sustain high-intensity activity (Moscatelli et al., 2020).

Ketogenic diets, often referred to as 'keto' are extremely high fat, typically resulting in a carbohydrate intake of 50 g per day or less. They were originally found to help those with hard-to-control epilepsy, and can still be used for this purpose. The aim is to push the body to convert fat into both fatty acids and ketones, and to use these as the main fuels for both brain and muscles.

The proposal is that consuming a high fat/keto diet will increase the availability and the use of fats as a fuel and preserve glycogen stores. Unfortunately, this results in a slower resynthesis of ATP which can't meet the energy demand in high-intensity movement – which dance involves. Also, high-intensity exercise suppresses the rate of fat metabolism, so there are less fatty acids actually available as fuel for muscles (Zajac et al., 2014). Also burning fat, because it uses more oxygen, increases the risk that the brain will not receive adequate energy supplies.

There are potential side effects of a very high fat/low carb ketogenic diet including low blood glucose levels, dehydration and kidney stones (Hartman & Vining, 2007) – far from ideal for a dancer. The diet also requires significant supplementation with vitamin and minerals due to the limited range of foods eaten. Add to this the reported poor concentration and low mood that can occur with very low carb intakes as the brain favours carb not fat as a fuel, and there can be no recommendation for a high fat or keto diet for any dancer undertaking high-intensity dance activity.

VI Resources

Digestion and Absorption of Lipids|LibreTexts Nutrition (lumenlearning. com).
Extra Virgin Olive Oil and Athletes – Sports Dietitians Australia (SDA).

VII Learning outcomes

After reading this chapter the reader should be able to:

1 State examples of the roles fats play within the body.
2 Summarise the roles omega-3 play in health and well-being and the challenges of meeting requirements.
3 Explain why dancers are advised not to follow a high-fat meal plan.
4 Discuss food choices that will help dancers meet goals for dietary fats.

References

Burdge, G.C., Jones, A.E. and Wootton, S.A. (2002) Eicosapentaenoic and docos-apentaenoic acids are the principal products of α-linolenic acid metabolism in young men, *British Journal of Nutrition*, 88(4), pp.355–363.

Burdge, G.C. and Wootton, S.A. (2002) Conversion of α-linolenic acid to eicosapen-taenoic, docosapentaenoic and docosahexaenoic acids in young women, *British Journal of Nutrition*, 88(4), pp.411–420.

Carriere, F. et al. (1993) Secretion and contribution to lipolysis of gastric and pan-creatic lipases during a test meal in humans, *Gastroenterology*, 105(3), pp.876–888.

Corder, K.E. et al. (2016) Effects of short-term docosahexaenoic acid supplemen-tation on markers of inflammation after eccentric strength exercise in women, *Journal of Sports Science & Medicine*, 15(1), pp.176.

Dowhan, W. (1997). The role of phospholipids in cell function. *Advances in Lipobi-ology*, 2, pp.79–107.

Hamosh, M. (1990) Lingual and gastric lipases, *Nutrition* (Burbank, Los Angeles County, Calif.), 6(6), pp.421–428.

Hartman, A.L. and Vining, E.P. (2007) Clinical aspects of the ketogenic diet, *Epilepsia*, 48(1), pp.31–42.

Jouris, K.B., McDaniel, J.L. and Weiss, E.P. (2011) The effect of omega-3 fatty acid supplementation on the inflammatory response to eccentric strength exercise, *Journal of Sports Science & Medicine*, 10(3), pp.432.

Lewis, N.A. et al. (2020) Are there benefits from the use of fish oil supplements in athletes? A systematic review, *Advances in Nutrition*, 11(5), pp.1300–1314.

Moscatelli, F. et al. (2020) Ketogenic diet and sport performance, *Sport Mont*, 18(1), pp.91–94.

Thomas, D.T., Erdman, K.A. and Burke, L.M. (2016) American college of sports medicine joint position statement. Nutrition and athletic performance, *Medicine and Science in Sports and Exercise*, 48(3), pp.543–568.

Zajac, A. et al. (2014) The effects of a ketogenic diet on exercise metabolism and physical performance in off-road cyclists, *Nutrients*, 6(7), pp.2493–2508.

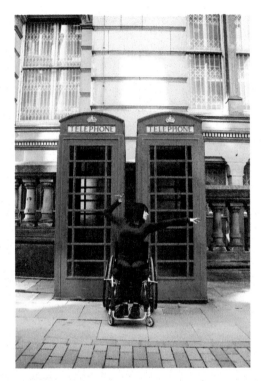

Photo 7.1 Dancers perform in different conditions: matching fluid intake to the environmental conditions allows optimal hydration.

Credit: Photo courtesy of Dani Bower photography

7   Hydration for stamina and performance optimisation

Contents

Key points for staying hydrated

Challenges to hydration	Practical points
Fluid is lost overnight and during the day even without exercise	Aim to be hydrated before training/rehearsals/performances start: drink when you get up and regularly through classes, rehearsals and performances
Sweating results in additional fluid losses, and this can impair performance	Aim to stay hydrated over the day: keep fluid losses below 2% body weight: check occasionally to make sure
The recommended replacement of 1.5 × sweat loss could mean an intake of over 1 l per class	Check your water bottle is large enough: 750–1,000 ml is more useful than 500 ml
As exercise intensity increases stomach emptying and digestion of fluids slows down and this can be a challenge to hydration	Drink small amounts regularly: 150–200 ml every 20–30 minutes: the body can tolerate 300 –1,000 ml per hour though you may need to build up amounts over time: training the gut is possible

(Continued)

DOI: 10.4324/9781003219002-7

Key points for staying hydrated

Challenges to hydration	Practical points
Sweat is mainly water but does contain some electrolytes. Because exercise is using fuel it is helping to replace all of these components when possible	Choice: drinks with up to 8% carb and some electrolytes are useful (but spillages need to be avoided in the studio)
During performances opportunities to drink may be limited, but rarely for longer than 45 minutes	Being able to tolerate up to 45 minutes without drinking is useful for performance situations. In training teachers need to liaise with the dancers to agree when 'fluid free' training is undertaken, so that dancers are not avoiding fluids unnecessarily

I Introduction

Your body works best when it contains the volume of water that is normal and adequate for you: neither too much nor too little. This state of being in fluid balance is known as euhydration. The body can tolerate some minor fluctuations which normally occur, but as more major fluctuations occur, mechanisms kick in to try and correct the imbalance. If you over drink, your kidneys will filter the excess water which will be sent to them in your blood and you will produce more urine, which will also usually be more dilute. This will result in more trips to the bathroom. If fluid losses are greater than replacement then you start to become dehydrated. Dehydration refers to the process of losing body water and leads to reduced levels of body water known as hypohydration. Urine production falls in dehydration. It is worth noting at this point that exercise also reduces urine production as the kidneys receive less blood flow and the muscles receive more blood flow to allow oxygen and nutrients to reach the working muscles. Your body will pick up the fact that fluid levels are dropping and will signal thirst, which aims to get you to drink and correct the imbalance. The amount, composition and timing of drinks can all impact on how quickly you rehydrate and all of this will be discussed shortly.

II What the body needs fluid for

1   *Core temperature regulation: preventing overheating*
     When you dance, or undertake other physical activity, heat is produced as a byproduct of the exercise. Research has shown that the human body will not function optimally, if heat produced is not dissipated: our bodies function best at a core temperature of around 36–37°C (96.8–98.6°F), above and below this temperature many essential body processes work less well, and at extremes, dance will not be possible. It is vital to get rid of much of the heat produced in exercising to

avoid overheating and compromising body functions. Sweating is the main way humans dissipate heat. In addition to heat produced from dance, heavy costumes, hot stage lighting and hot environmental conditions can all add to the challenges to dancers' temperature regulation. Temperature regulation can be an additional challenge to dancers with some disabilities: those with spinal cord injuries are at particular risk (Price & Trbovich, 2018) and may face a particular challenge to stay hydrated. Additionally, dancers who face mobility challenges accessing toilet facilities may be tempted to drink less to reduce urine formation. If this applies to you, you are encouraged to speak with relevant individuals to see what can be done to optimise the situation for your specific circumstances.

2   *Maintaining body water content and limiting fluctuations*
Your body is about 60% water. Water is the major component of blood, and muscle has a high water content of around 75% (Lorenzo et al., 2019). Even fat cells contain around 10% water. If water is lost but not replaced, then dehydration begins.

Water is lost daily from the body in a number of ways:

1   In urine: amount variable, but around 800–2,000 ml per 24 hours, is normal. 700 ml or less in 24 hours is likely to be too little to excrete waste products. Being at altitude or in a cold environment also increases urine production.
2   Fluid is lost when breathing out, as the air in the lungs needs to have a high water content and this moist air is then expelled from the body. This loss is greater at altitude when the air has a lower moisture content. Estimates of fluid loss from breath are 2.7 ml/min from breath for hard exercise in dry (20% humidity) air though only 0.8 ml/min from breath for hard exercise in high (80%) humidity (Maughan et al., 2007). As a guide you will be losing at least 50 ml water per hour in breath. Although breath losses will be less when the air is humid it is important to note that sweat losses will be higher (Maughan et al., 2012). Being at altitude will increase fluid losses from breath which needs to be considered if you are temporarily or permanently or in a location at altitude, e.g., Denver, Colorado.
3   Fluid is lost from the bowels in faeces (stools). This will be increased if diarrhoea is experienced. Vomiting will also increase fluid losses.
4   Fluid is lost from the skin even when at rest. This will increase in activity when sweating is the main form of heat loss for humans.

Together the fluid lost from the bowel, skin and breath in health and at rest is around 500 ml (around a pint) per day, to be added to urine losses, plus additional sweat losses in dance and other activities.

III   Dehydration and its impact on the dancer's health and performance

What is dehydration?

Dehydration is when body water levels fall below normal. This should result in thirst, but this is hard to measure. If you are thirsty then responding to this is almost always a good plan (occasionally people get used to drinking excessive amounts yet still feel thirsty; this needs to be checked out medically). Responding to thirst is now recognised as the best way to stay hydrated. Your body can tolerate a small amount of dehydration and still function effectively providing the fluid lost is replaced promptly to prevent more severe dehydration as activity continues.

Blood or urine tests give the most detail which allows researchers to identify the consequences of dehydration. However, research with athletes and dancers involving blood tests and urine analysis isn't always practical, but there is a much easier method that is accepted as valid across a short time period (hours not days). This is to check your body weight immediately before and straight after exercise, wearing dry clothing for both measurements and emptying the bladder before each weighing. As 1 l of water weighs 1 kg, it is simple to identify whether approximately enough fluid has been taken in to balance losses, particularly those from sweating. This is discussed in more detail shortly. Research on the effects of dehydration can be hard to identify as it is difficult to study for a few reasons, one of these being that people vary in their response to dehydration. Overall dehydration is known to reduce performance (James et al., 2019).

The consequences of dehydration

If your fluid intake is inadequate to replace fluid losses, and your body water content starts to drop there are a number of serious consequences that will impact on your ability to dance. These include blood becoming more viscous (thicker). It will then become less efficient at transporting gases, nutrients and waste products and can then result in cardiovascular strain. You will use increased amounts of your glycogen stores for the same workload and will have altered metabolic and central nervous system (CNS) function in the case of dehydration (Thomas et al., 2016). From research there is growing knowledge on the impact of different levels of dehydration, using short-term per cent body weight loss as the scale for identifying the consequences. To put this into context, the weight changes that would be seen at different levels are:

For a 50-kg female: 10% dehydration would be a 5 kg very rapid weight drop and 2% dehydration would be a 1 kg weight drop.

For a 70-kg male: 10% dehydration would be 7 kg while 2% translates to 1.4 kg (Maughan, 2003, Sawka et al., 2007, Sawka et al., 2015). All of the changes in body weight below are rapid, over a period of hours to a few days maximum.

- One to two per cent body weight loss should trigger thirst without impairing your ability to dance.
- Two per cent body weight loss: this level of loss is widely used as the cut-off point where impairment to exercise starts and as the cut-off for the start of being in a state of hypohydration.
- Four to eight per cent body weight loss: some elite athletes are able to perform well but most athletes and dancers will see a significant drop in performance, together with fatigue and an increasing risk of dizziness, muscle cramps, headaches and feeling generally unwell.
- Five per cent body weight loss: impact on the ability to concentrate.
- Twelve per cent body weight loss: extreme dehydration. This is very unlikely to occur outside of severe medical conditions resulting in fluid loss or a complete lack of access to food and fluid for several days. The body is likely to go into shock, with organs shutting down, and there is a risk of death above this.

As dehydration increases the impacts are more serious: 2–7% dehydration causes reduced endurance capacity by highly variable amounts: the impact has been shown to be between 7% and 60% reduction. Skill level has also been reported to be reduced by dehydration (Maughan & Shirreffs, 2010). For dancers, this could translate into struggling to perform intricate footwork or precise movements accurately.

The impact of dehydration on exercise performance is likely to be greater if you are both dehydrated and in hot conditions: as air temperature increases the impact of dehydration on performance. There is also a health consequence to not meeting your fluid needs: in the long-term chronic dehydration can increase the risk of kidney stones.

Composition of sweat and why it matters

Sweat is mainly composed of water and electrolytes. Electrolytes are substances that conduct electricity when dissolved in water and are essential for human health. There are also traces of water-soluble vitamins lost in sweat, but these losses are unlikely to impact on your well-being. Urea (a waste product of protein metabolism) and lactic acid are also lost in sweat, together with small amounts of uric acid and creatinine (Mickelson & Keys, 1943). The main electrolytes lost are sodium, chloride and potassium, but small amounts of others including magnesium, calcium, copper and zinc are also lost (Montain et al., 2007). Some dancers will lose more electrolytes in sweat than others. Sodium sweat losses can be very varied, from 10 to 90 mmol/l, though typically around 40–60 mmol/l. This is likely to be a significant proportion of your daily intake. Your body does have some ability to control the amount of salt lost so that you don't lose excessive amounts, and many dancers even with several hours dancing per day find water is a suitable drink. Potassium losses in sweat are typically under 5 mmol/l, which is a small proportion of a day's intake. Magnesium losses are around 2–3 mmol/l, which is likely to be a higher proportion of a day's typical intake than potassium, but almost certainly less than sodium. Calcium losses in sweat are relatively small compared to normal intakes. Although food can provide these electrolytes, there are situations where using drinks with salts can be useful. Practical advice on this is given later in this chapter in Section III and Chapter 8.

IV Identifying and calculating your fluid needs

Do I need to calculate how much fluid I need? Can't I just rely on thirst?

Some people have a good sense of thirst, and research has shown that these people, even when taking part in exercise, are able to pretty much meet their fluid requirements as long as they have access to suitable amounts of suitable fluids while they exercise. Others have a less good sense of thirst and may go several hours without taking on board any liquid, even when exercising. If you are unsure which group you fit into then it's useful to pay particular attention to how much you drink over a period of up to seven days. Taking note of your urine output is useful too: how often you pee; is it a small or large volume. Your bladder capacity is around 300–600 ml, although at night it may cope with a slightly larger volume. Precisely, 200 ml is a small amount of urine to pass at one time, and 400–500+ml is a large volume. Also check the colour: how dark or pale it is. Dark yellow urine will have been formed when the body has not had adequate fluid going through the kidneys. And urine volume will be smaller if there is limited fluid intake. As urine forms over a few hours, the colour and volume are reflective of your state of hydration since you last passed urine. If you have just drunk a good volume of fluid and then immediately empty your bladder, the urine will not yet reflect the improved intake.

The aim is for urine to be pale, straw coloured and to pass good volumes every few hours. If you are managing this it suggests you are doing well with your fluid intake and most likely meeting your requirements (Figure 7.1).

Making notes of amounts drunk and the timings you tend to drink more and less can identify whether there are good and less good times/situations and allow you to plan changes if you are not meeting your fluid needs.

Fluid balance and fluid losses: how fluid can be gained

To get a better idea of the causes of fluid fluctuations in your body it can be useful to think about both sides of the fluid balance equation: fluid out and fluid in. There are three main ways the body gains water and four main ways fluid is lost, which are shown in Table 7.1.

Replacing sweat losses

Sweat rates have been shown to be very variable: research reports evidence of approx. 800–1,200 ml/hour for males and 400–600 ml per hour for

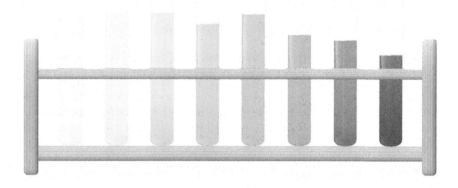

Figure 7.1 Darker urine colour and reduced volume indicate increased levels of dehydration since last bladder emptying.
Credit: Peter Hermes Furian/Shutterstock

Table 7.1 Fluid lost and gained by the body

Water lost from your body	*Water gained by your body*
In breath	0.6 ml water produced per gram of carb metabolised
In urine	1.1 ml water produced per gram of fat metabolised
In stools	From food: variable amount: depends on food choices: cucumber is 97% water, crackers just 5% water
From skin as sweat	From all drinks (except alcohol which results overall in loss not gain)

females, though there are wide variations between individuals even when the air temperature, humidity and workload are the same (Wyndham et al., 1965; Burke & Hawley, 1997).

Your rate of sweating at a particular dance intensity is partly genetic, but it will be influenced by how well you are acclimatised to the conditions and your training. Some disabilities can impact on sweat rates, and wheelchair dancers in particular may benefit from individual advice on fluids. If you are suddenly dancing in a hotter climate than normal, it will feel harder for the first few days while your body adjusts and increases your sweat rate to disperse more heat. If you are familiar with the dance work you are undertaking you will perform it more economically with less heat produced

(Sawka et al., 2007). It is useful to remember that effective sweating is where sweat evaporates and removes heat from the body – so you don't see the sweat being lost and may be unaware of it particularly in colder conditions. Sweat that doesn't evaporate because it stays on/in clothing or drips off the body is also fluid that has been lost: but without getting rid of any heat – and the extra losses still need to be replaced.

Estimating sweat losses from dance

Measuring sweat losses accurately requires equipment not readily available outside research laboratories. The good news is that there is a simple, practical way of estimating whether you currently meet your fluid needs, which is to check your body weight on a reliable scale before and after dancing.

- For this you will need to be in dry clothing before the class/rehearsal and have similar dry clothing to put on afterwards.
- Both weights need to be done with an empty bladder.
- Fluid drunk in class/rehearsal needs to be recorded.

Example: dancer A weighs 63.5 kg before a 1.5-hour class. After class, they weigh 62.8 kg. During class they drank 300 ml. Weight loss of 0.7 kg = 0.7 l (700 ml). As they drank 0.3 l but still lost 0.7 kg they needed around 1 l of fluid.

Over the next few weeks, the dancer plans to: gradually increase the amount they drink in this class. They tend to find they feel bloated when drinking, but they know that the gut can be trained to manage larger amounts of both food and fluid. While 400–800 ml per hour will be enough for many dancers, if they are drinking to thirst and also taking in some fluids from food, up to 1,000 ml per hour can be absorbed with practice. If this amount is needed, it is best spread over the hour into at least three drinks. For those with back-to-back classes or rehearsals, it is good practice to try and keep up with fluid intake during classes as far as is practical, so that breaks can be used to focus on nutrition and being ready for the next class.

Is it always necessary to drink during dance activities?

If you are hydrated at the start of class/rehearsal/performance and if it is for no more than an hour, and also the only physical activity you are doing that day, then it is not essential to try and take on board any fluids during that hour. But this is rarely the case for to most dancers, as, whether students or professionals, the amount of dance and additional training is well over an hour per day, and typically classes and rehearsals run back to back. For this reason, it is important to drink fluids during classes and rehearsals, as well as performances. Timing and advice on this is given below.

Hydration: pre dance strategies

- It sounds obvious – and it is, but not always easy: arrive to start your dance schedule hydrated. For some this is straightforward. If you have no problem having breakfast and fluid in the morning, and then eating and drinking regularly until physical activity starts, whether it's warm up and class, a gym visit, or maybe a run or swim, then you will be able to start hydrated. But some dancers struggle to eat and drink first thing and are likely to arrive dehydrated. If this is you, your body can adapt, as long as you start with small amounts, around 100–200 ml of the fluid you find easiest, and work towards at least 200–300 ml at least 30 minutes before you start asking your body to work physically. Many dancers have found that over time they are able to not just make these changes but also to feel the benefits of the new strategies.
- If you are unsure if you are hydrated before any dance activity, but particularly assessments, exams or performances, there is a quick way to make sure: drink around 250–500 ml depending on your body weight (5–7 ml/kg per body weight) at least four hours before you are due to dance. If you don't need to pass urine over the next two hours, or the urine is dark or highly concentrated, you should slowly drink more: around 150–350 ml (3–5 ml/kg) about two hours before the event. Using an isotonic drink or a drink with salts may help retain the water (, Thomas et al., 2016).

Hydration – strategies during dance and other physical activity

- Drinking large amounts at one time is less effective for hydration than smaller amounts more regularly: the kidneys will sense a large amount of additional fluid and will begin to excrete it. The most effective strategy is to drink 200–400 ml every 20–30 minutes during moderate-to-high intensity dance. If the pace is slower, then it's fine to drink a little less – and always rely on thirst to guide you if you can.
- Checking that your water bottle is large enough: a 500-ml bottle is only useful for short classes at low intensity unless you are able to refill it regularly.
- Aim to keep up with your fluid requirements/thirst if at all possible: research has shown that to restore fluid balance requires taking in more than 100% of fluid lost. The recommendation is to take in 1.25–1.5 ml for every 1 ml lost (Thomas et al., 2016).
- General health and well-being point: it is best not to share water bottles. Remember viruses can be spread by an infected person before they feel unwell. Dancers work in close proximity to others; viruses as well as bacteria can therefore spread easily. Avoiding sharing drinks is one way to reduce the risks as far as is possible.

Hydration – strategies after dance and other physical activity

- If your dance workload resulted in higher sweat losses than usual you may not have managed to keep up with your requirements. Prioritise fluid intake before your next dance session. This may mean drinking and then eating around 30 minutes later, or drinking and eating at the same time. The second option can lead to feeling particularly full in the short term, but rehydration and refuelling are both necessary. If you have foods with a high water content, such as vegetables/salad/fruit these will supply some water – on average around 80%, which is a valuable contribution to your intake.
- If your diet is high in either salt and/or protein you will need additional fluid to excrete the salt and/or the metabolites of protein. Consider whether either or both are needed and reduce salt gradually if possible. Take particular note of thirst and respond to this. If your sense of thirst isn't great, then focus on having a little extra every time you drink.
- Make sure you rehydrate before you drink alcohol or large amounts of caffeine, as these will worsen dehydration and recovery from exercise.

Hydration strategies in a heat wave or when travelling to hotter climates

- If the air temperature increases, or for example, you travel to an area that is much hotter than you are used to, your body will increase sweat rates to minimise increases in core temperature. Ensure you drink enough regularly to match increased sweat rates – take note of urine output and increase fluids if volume decreases and/or colour darkens.
- Heat adaptation takes a few days and any physical work load will feel harder until the body adapts by increasing sweat rates and fluid intake. Aim to reduce dance workload in the first two to three days in a hotter climate.
- Flying dehydrates due to the dry air in the plane at altitude. Particularly on long-haul flights, make sure you are drinking slightly more than you would on a rest day at home and avoid or limit alcohol. If you do drink alcohol while flying then aim to also drink an additional 150 ml water per unit of alcohol.

Hydration strategies for assessments, exams and other infrequent dance events

When exams or other infrequent events loom, the best strategy is the one you have practiced: it is unwise to try unfamiliar foods/drinks/amounts of drinks in a situation where you want to be at your best.

This principle does also apply to performances, for example, an overseas tour, with the added factor that drinks can only be taken when you are off stage for long enough. During the rehearsal process start to research fluid choice options, and any changes to opportunities for drinking and practice as best you can so you have an idea how you can best stay hydrated when you get to the performances.

The risks of drinking too much water

While it is essential to avoid dehydration, overdrinking resulting in overhydration will not improve performance and in fact excess fluid can be both uncomfortable and impact negatively on health and performance. Symptoms of overhydration include nausea or vomiting, a headache, tiredness, muscle cramps and at its most severe confusion and seizures. These will be caused by low levels of electrolytes, particularly sodium (hyponatraemia) (Noakes, 2003). As a rough rule of thumb, if you are a female dancer drinking over 4 l per day, or a male dancer drinking over 5.5 l (unless in extreme heat conditions) check how this fluid is spread out over the day, check your fluid losses in classes/rehearsals (see weight difference method above), make a note of urine output and consider reducing your intake gradually. If you check your weight before and after a class or rehearsal and you have gained weight, then you have most likely drunk more than needed (unless you started dehydrated) and are advised to gradually reduce your intake until you are in balance. Current recommendations are to drink to thirst over the day to avoid overdrinking. And if thirst doesn't meet requirements, then to use the guidance above to make sure you do have enough fluid but avoid overdrinking.

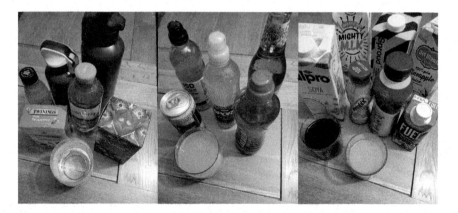

Photo 7.2 Examples of hypotonic, isotonic and hypertonic drinks.

V Fluid choices – hypotonic, isotonic and hypertonic drinks

Drinks are typically divided into three categories according to how they compare with body fluids. The relationship between the drink and body fluids has an impact on how fast the drink is absorbed and, therefore, how useful it is likely to be during dance.

Hypotonic fluids contain fewer particles then body fluids and are absorbed relatively quickly. They will have an osmolality (number of particles in 1 kg of water) of 50–270 mOsmol/kg (EFSA, 2011). Hypotonic fluids include water, sugar-free drinks and those drinks with less than 4 g carbohydrate per 100 ml. Water has the advantage that it is most easily available and is usually permissible in dance studios when other drinks may not be allowed due to the risk of damage to flooring.

Isotonic fluids contain similar numbers of particles to body fluids. If isotonic fluids have the concentration of particles measured, they will have an osmolality of 270–330 mOsmol/kg (EFSA, 2011). Typically they will contain

Table 7.2 Advantages and disadvantages of fluid choices

Type of fluid	Examples	Advantages	Disadvantages	Notes
Hypotonic	Water, herbal teas, sugar-free drinks, low-sugar drinks	Absorbed quickly, water is cheap, easily accessible, safe and can be taken into most dance spaces	Will not replace energy used, may not replace electrolytes	All water is suitable, though fizzy water may cause gas problems
Isotonic: 4–8 g carb per 100 ml plus some electrolytes	Many sports drinks – check the nutrition label, homemade isotonic drinks (see recipe section)	Absorbed quickly, will supplement energy levels and replace minerals	The energy is from carb with few other nutrients Possible impact on dental health	Rinse the mouth with water after an isotonic drink to protect teeth
Hypertonic	Milk, protein shakes, fruit juice, most soft drinks (cola, some lemonades), energy drinks	Can supply carbohydrate and other nutrients	Absorbed slowly, not useful when quick rehydration is needed.	
Hydration powders/ Electrolyte supplements added to water	Electrolyte tablets and powders made by sports nutrition companies	Can replace electrolytes as well as fluid. Easily transportable	Will not replace energy used. Information on absorption rates lacking. May not have the optimal balance of electrolytes	Not advised for those under 16 years old. Some contain caffeine.

4–8 g carbohydrate per 100 ml, plus sodium, potassium and possibly other electrolytes such as calcium or magnesium. Isotonic sports drinks may contain additional vitamins, typically from the B group.

Hypertonic fluids contain more particles than body fluids, for example, a sugar content of 9+ g per 100 ml, higher levels of salts, or other particles for example, proteins or fats.

Table 7.2 summarises the different fluid options for hydration and their advantages and disadvantages for the dancer.

Milk and milk alternatives as recovery drinks

Although absorbed more slowly than hypotonic or isotonic drinks, there is evidence that milk or flavoured milk can be useful as a recovery drink as it can supply good-quality protein, carbohydrate and electrolytes. Plant milk substitutes can contribute to carbohydrate, but many are low in protein, although soy, pea and some brands of oat drink will have protein closest to that in cow's milk.

Chocolate milk has been used in research with athletes and cyclists to aid recovery after training has finished, with the aim of enhancing the next performance and could also be useful for dancers.

For those following a vegan diet, the best option is likely to be using a good-quality protein shake (you are advised to check that any products you use have been tested via the www.informed-sport testing system to minimise the risk of contaminants).

Having a milk-based drink after harder dance sessions when there is time to absorb this (at least an hour break or at the end of the dance schedule) can be a useful way to start recovery and refuelling for the next day.

Fluid choices

Drinks to rehydrate before/during/after shorter/less intense training/performance	Drinks before/during training/performance to support both hydration and carb levels	Drinks useful after intense training/performance to support muscle recovery and replace carbs
Water (consider adding electrolytes)	Isotonic drinks – homemade (see recipe section) or bought	Milkshake/smoothie
Water flavoured with a small amount of cordial		Protein shake that includes carb, typically 3:1 carb: protein content (grams)
Low-sugar drinks		
Fruit teas/herbal teas		

Caffeine

Caffeine is a substance that can be found in many drinks, whether hypotonic, isotonic or hypertonic. Historically, there has been much criticism of drinks with caffeine with concern they will result in increased fluids losses in urine and will increase the risk of dehydration compared with other drinks. The current consensus is that small amounts of caffeine, up to 180 mg per day (Thomas et al., 2016), will not impact on urine output. This amount could be found in one strong cup of coffee, or two cups of average coffee, or two to three cups of tea. In practice, dancers who are used to including caffeine in their diet are likely to tolerate three to four cups of normal-strength tea/coffee per day without any impact on hydration. As caffeine does have a role in increasing alertness it can have some benefits and dancers may consider using it to help performance. See Chapter 8 for more information and caffeine content of drinks. Energy drinks usually have a high caffeine content so dancers are advised to check the amount before drinking and evaluate whether the benefits of caffeine will outweigh any possible disadvantage of increased dehydration.

VI A quick note about alcohol

There are unfortunately no benefits from alcohol when it comes to hydration. There are also many disadvantages to performance. Alcohol dehydrates: it is estimated that each unit of alcohol will cause 100 ml of water to be lost from the body (Eggleton, 1942). The effect of beer at 4–5% alcohol does not seem to have a significant impact on hydration, although consuming alcohol even at 4% concentration seems to slow recovery from dehydration after exercise (Shirreffs & Maughan, 1997). If alcohol is taken instead of carbohydrate after exercise glycogen repletion will be reduced (Burke et al., 2003).

Research suggests that alcohol consumption decreases the use of glucose and amino acids by skeletal muscles in exercise which will adversely affect energy supply and impair metabolic processes during exercise (El-Sayed et al., 2005). If alcohol is consumed before dance, it will impair central nervous system function depending on the amount taken, resulting in reductions in cognitive function and motor skill, as well as behavioural changes that may have adverse effects on performance (Shirreffs & Maughan, 2006).

VII Resources

Tyler, C.J. (2019). *Maximising Performance in Hot Environments: A Problem-Based Learning Approach*. Routledge.

Fluids and Hydration|U.S. Anti-Doping Agency (USADA).

Maughan, R.J., Watson, P., Cordery, P.A., Walsh, N.P., Oliver, S.J., Dolci, A., Rodriguez-Sanchez, N., and Galloway, S.D. (2016). A randomized trial to assess the potential of different beverages to affect hydration status: Development of a beverage hydration index. *The American Journal of Clinical Nutrition.* 103(3), pp. 717–723.

VIII Learning outcomes

After reading this chapter the reader should be able to:

1   Explain the consequences to the dancer of becoming dehydrated.
2   List strategies to prevent dehydration before and during dance and other physical activity.
3   Explain the differences between hypotonic, isotonic and hypertonic drinks.
4   State suitable drinks for use during and after dance and other physical activity.

References

Burke, L.M. et al. (2003) Effect of alcohol intake on muscle glycogen storage after prolonged exercise, *Journal of Applied Physiology*, 95(3), pp.983–990.

Burke, L.M. and Hawley, J.A. (1997) Fluid balance in team sports, *Sports Medicine*, 24(1), pp.38–54.

EFSA Panel on Dietetic Products, Nutrition and Allergies (NDA) (2011) Scientific opinion on the substantiation of health claims related to carbohydrate-electrolyte solutions and reduction in rated perceived exertion/effort during exercise (ID 460, 466, 467, 468), enhancement of water absorption during exercise (ID 314, 315, 316, 317, 319, 322, 325, 332, 408, 465, 473, 1168, 1574, 1593, 1618, 4302, 4309), and maintenance of endurance performance (ID 466, 469) pursuant to article 13 (1) of regulation (EC) no 1924/2006, *EFSA Journal*, 9(6), p.2211.

Eggleton, M.G. (1942) The diuretic action of alcohol in man 1, *The Journal of Physiology*, 101(2), pp.172–191.

El-Sayed, M.S., Ali, N. and Ali, Z.E. (2005) Interaction between alcohol and exercise, *Sports Medicine*, 35(3), pp.257–269.

James, L.J. et al. (2019) Does hypohydration really impair endurance performance? Methodological considerations for interpreting hydration research, *Sports Medicine*, 49(2), pp.103–114.

Lorenzo, I., Serra-Prat, M. and Yébenes, J.C. (2019) The role of water homeostasis in muscle function and frailty: A review, *Nutrients*, 11(8), p.1857.

Maughan, R.J. (2003) Impact of mild dehydration on wellness and on exercise performance, *European Journal of Clinical Nutrition*, 57(2), pp.S19–S23.

Maughan, R.J. and Shirreffs, S.M. (2010) Dehydration and rehydration in competitive sport, *Scandinavian Journal of Medicine & Science in Sports*, 20, pp.40–47.

Maughan, R.J., Otani, H. and Watson, P. (2012) Influence of relative humidity on prolonged exercise capacity in a warm environment, *European Journal of Applied Physiology*, 112(6), pp.2313–2321.

Maughan, R.J., Shirreffs, S.M. and Leiper, J.B. (2007) Errors in the estimation of hydration status from changes in body mass, *Journal of Sports Sciences*, 25(7), pp.797–804.

Mickelsen, O. and Keys, A. (1943) The composition of sweat, with special reference to the vitamins, *Journal of Biological Chemistry*, 149(2), pp.479–490.

Montain, S.J., Cheuvront, S.N. and Lukaski, H.C. (2007) Sweat mineral-element responses during 7 h of exercise-heat stress, *International Journal of Sport Nutrition and Exercise Metabolism*, 17(6), pp.574–582.

Noakes, T.D. (2003) Overconsumption of fluids by athletes, *Bmj*, 327(7407), pp.113–114.

Price, M.J. and Trbovich, M. (2018) Thermoregulation following spinal cord injury, in *Anonymous Handbook of Clinical Neurology*, Elsevier, pp. 799–820.

Sawka, M.N. et al. (2007) American college of sports medicine position stand. exercise and fluid replacement, *Medicine and Science in Sports and Exercise*, 39(2), pp.377–390.

Sawka, M.N., Cheuvront, S.N. and Kenefick, R.W. (2015) Hypohydration and human performance: Impact of environment and physiological mechanisms, *Sports Medicine*, 45(1), pp.51–60.

Shirreffs, S.M. and Maughan, R.J. (1997) Restoration of fluid balance after exercise-induced dehydration: Effects of alcohol consumption, *Journal of Applied Physiology*, 83(4), pp.1152–1158.

Shirreffs, S.M. and Maughan, R.J. (2006) The effect of alcohol on athletic performance, *Current Sports Medicine Reports*, 5(4), pp.192–196.

Thomas, D. T., Erdman, K. A., & Burke, L. M. (2016). Position of the Academy of Nutrition and Dietetics, Dietitians of Canada, and the American College of Sports Medicine: Nutrition and athletic performance. *Journal of the Academy of Nutrition and Dietetics*, *116*(3), pp.501–528.

Wyndham, C.H., Morrison, J.F. and Williams, C.G. (1965) Heat reactions of male and female Caucasians, *Journal of Applied Physiology*, 20(3), pp.357–364.

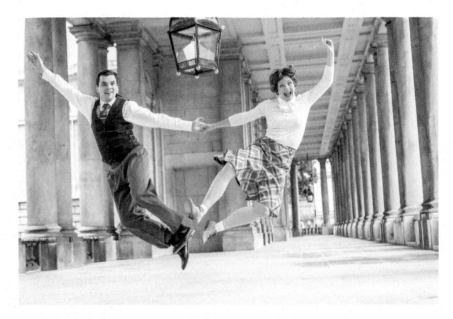

Photo 8.1 'Nutrition supplements can be useful, but nutrients from food are the
        priority to fuel great dance performances'.

Credit: Photo courtesy of Helen Rimmell

8 Supplements to support health and performance (to supplement food not replace it)

Contents

I Dietary supplements and ergogenic aids

Introduction

'Dietary supplements' is a term that covers a wide variety of substances. The US government defines supplements as: 'products taken by mouth that contain a "dietary ingredient." Dietary ingredients include vitamins, minerals, amino acids, and herbs or botanicals, as well as other substances that can be used to supplement the diet'. In the International Olympic Committee (IOC) consensus statement on dietary supplements and the high-performance athlete (Maughan et al., 2018), supplements are defined as: 'a food, food component, nutrient, or non-food compound that is purposefully ingested in addition to the habitually consumed diet with the aim of achieving a specific health and/or performance benefit'. This definition acknowledges the dual role products can have, supporting health and/or performance.

Dietary supplements come in many forms, including tablets, capsules, powders, bars, and liquids. Dietary supplements that dancers may consider taking, or be taking, include vitamins and/or minerals, protein powders or drinks, carbohydrate gels/powders, substances such as creatine, glucosamine, turmeric, and concentrated extracts from foods such as beetroot juice. The difference between a food product and a dietary supplement can sometimes be hard to identify, particularly if the supplement is an extract of a food. Supplements can be a single nutrient/compound or a combination of two or more nutrients/compounds.

DOI: 10.4324/9781003219002-8

'Ergogenic aids' have been defined as:

> A technique or substance used for the purpose of enhancing perfor-
> mance. Ergogenic aids have been classified as nutritional, pharma-
> cologic, physiologic, or psychologic and range from use of accepted
> techniques such as carbohydrate loading to illegal and unsafe ap-
> proaches such as anabolic-androgenic steroid use.
>
> (Thein et al., 1995)

As this is a nutrition book, nutritional ergogenic aids, rather than any other
categories of ergogenic aid will be explored here.

Not all supplements are ergogenic aids; some supplements are taken only
to enhance health rather than performance. Not all ergogenic aids are supplements, as some have no obvious health benefits. Examples of ergogenic
aids are amino acids in high doses, caffeine, peppermint, tart cherry juice
and beetroot juice. As with supplements, they may be a single compound or
a combination.

Are supplements and ergogenic aids safe to take?

Although dancers have greater nutrient needs when compared to the
general population, many dancers will neither need nor benefit from a
supplement – with the exception of vitamin D which is discussed in detail
in this chapter. There are some dancers who will benefit from specific supplements and this will also be explored. Weighing against the benefits are
also some risks. Supplements can be contaminated with substances that
are banned for athletes. Dancers are not drug tested as athletes are but
equally are dancers going to want to take unknown substances when they
are expected to be taking a specific nutrient or compound? There are also
many claims about supplements and ergogenic aids which may not stand
up to deeper investigation. In the first instance, if you do decide to take a
supplement or ergogenic aid, then checking it is drug tested is a good starting point. In the UK, for example, the organisation responsible for testing
nutritional supplements and ergogenic aids is Informed Sport (Sports Sup-
plements Certification | Informed Sport (wetestyoutrust.com)). In the USA,
it's currently NSF Certified for Sport (Supplement Risk and NSF Certified
for Sport®|USADA).

Australia uses Informed Sport and also HASTA (Home – HASTA).

Depending on where you are living there may be another testing system
for supplements which you have access to. If a supplement isn't under a testing programme, then it does pose a risk as to whether the content is what the
manufacturer claims.

Section II looks at whether you might need to consider taking a supplement to make sure you meet your nutritional requirements. To get the most
benefit from any ergogenic aid, firstly make sure you are getting all the nutrients you need. Once you are confident your nutrition is on track then ergogenic aids are worth considering. As dance workloads can vary, Table 8.1

Table 8.1 What's the best way to assess if an ergogenic aid might help your performance?

Information to check	What to look for in the answer
Has the product been tested?	Peer reviewed research, in a scientific journal.
Is the result of taking the product significant? Are side effects listed?	An effect that is worth the costs and possible risks of any side effects.
How many people have trialled the product?	Case studies of 1 person are of limited use. Large groups are best (over 50 participants), smaller numbers, 10–50 give more limited data but are typical in research.
Which activity group has it been tested in?	Tested in sports relevant to dance (e.g., team sports) or in dance.
Are the trial participants at a similar level of training and skill as you are?	Effects in a comparable group: using untrained participants can give different results.
Which age groups has it been tested on?	A group similar age to yourself.
Are the trials short or long term?	How quickly you might see any benefits.
Are there exact details of the research protocol used: for example, the product, dose and timing?	Details that would allow you to assess if it is relevant for you, and if so to potentially follow the same protocol.
How long can you take the product for?	Details of the length of time that is considered safe for taking the supplement.
Are there any medications or other supplements/ergogenic aids that can't be taken at the same time?	Any information on this topic to avoid unwanted consequences.

gives some starting points to help you assess and use ergogenic aids as safely and effectively as possible.

What are the pluses and minuses of supplements and ergogenic aids?

Dietary supplements are intended to do just that – increase the nutrient content of the diet. Whether this is either necessary or beneficial depends on many factors. The goal for most dancers is to get the majority, if not all, of almost all the nutrients they need from their daily meals and snacks, by following the guidelines in previous chapters to meet requirements for macro and micro nutrients. There is one main exception – vitamin D – which will be explored in detail below. If you are deficient in a nutrient and struggling to meet your needs from food then a supplement could help achieve this. But an overdose would not be helpful. If you are currently taking more than one supplement check carefully about any repetition of nutrients between supplements which could result in a dose well above normal requirements. For some nutrients, for example, some of the B vitamins, this is unlikely to cause a problem (although you may find urine becomes bright yellow!). For other nutrients, for example, vitamin C, a significant excess can have a laxative effect at high doses, and this effect could impact significantly on performance. A large dose of a single micronutrient can also cause problems, for example, iron, zinc and calcium share the same transport system, so a large dose of one may cause a deficiency in another. Unless prescribed at high dose for a reason, then 100% of the nutrient reference value (NRV) is enough.

Nutritional ergogenic aids are many and varied. Caffeine is probably the best known and has been used by many of the world's population for centuries as a stimulant to enhance performance, both physical and mental. Even this well-known ergogenic aid does have negative effects if used in high doses, resulting in symptoms including anxiety and restlessness if too much is taken.

II Do I need a supplement?

This is a great question, and one to which the answer will always be: 'it depends'. And what it depends on is a number of factors, which include:

- If you are vegetarian or vegan
- If you avoid any foods/food groups
- If you are able to get adequate sunlight exposure all year round
- If you have any medical condition(s) that alter your nutritional requirements
- If you are trying to conceive, are pregnant or breastfeeding
- If you are anaemic
- If you struggle to meet your energy or macronutrient requirements from food
- If medical tests reveal you have a deficiency that requires a supplement
- It's best if at all possible to get all the nutrients you need from food (and some drinks). But there can be times when this is difficult, and situations where supplements are advised.
- If your day-to-day food intake is limited in range and likely to be low in one or more macronutrients, you are best to focus on making changes to food as a priority, as food supplies more than just the basic nutrients – many foods have additional substances that are beneficial to health, even if not vitamins or minerals. Many supplements won't give as good an effect as is possible if your basic food plan is lacking. If you are concerned that you have a limited intake of micronutrients – maybe you eat very little fruit or vegetables/salad at the moment, maybe you are working towards including nuts, seeds and pulses and wholegrains – then taking a one per day multivitamin and mineral with around 100% of the NRV, of as many vitamins and minerals as possible would be a good strategy in the short term while you work on variety and adequacy. It's worth noting that while eating a varied diet is extremely unlikely to lead to any overdoses of micronutrients, this is not the case with supplements. There are a few exceptions with food, for example, pregnant women need to avoid

liver due to the high content of vitamin A in liver. Be particularly careful with high doses of chromium, iron, vitamin C, vitamin D, vitamin A and vitamin B6 from supplements as these can cause side effects. If you are concerned your diet is inadequate and may need supplementing due to your current circumstances, then assessment and advice by a dietitian experienced in working with dancers are advisable.

Will a Nutritional Supplement help me?

Question	Consideration
• Why do I need a supplement?	• If your requirements are likely to be greater than your intake from food then supplements can help.
• Do I have high nutrient needs?	• If there are specific reasons you have high nutrient needs, whether it's due to your workload or medical situation that mean you need more than others do then a supplement could be useful.
• Will a balanced diet meet my specific needs?	• Other than vitamin D, unless you are aware of any reason increasing your needs then a balanced dancers' diet should meet your needs.
• Is this supplement safe?	• Check with Informed Sport or local system.
• Are the benefits of the supplement based on reliable scientific evidence?	• This requires looking at the supplement claim(s) and checking the data they cite as evidence.
• How much have I researched about this particular supplement?	• Check you have enough information to make an informed decision: be aware one brand may have a different composition in a different country.
• Am I familiar with the brand?	• If the answer is no, the some background checking would be useful.
• Have studies found the supplement effective?	• If there are no studies on the brand you are looking at, your best option is to look for a comparable brand with some data.
• Is it potentially a waste of money?	• If you don't have clear reasons for taking then your money is likely better spent on food.
• Do I think this supplement is going to make my goals reality?	• Be realistic about how any supplement can help – if it will correct a nutrient deficiency then you may see significant changes in performance, otherwise this is unlikely.
• Does this supplement interact with other supplements or medications?	• Check on any medication you take for any supplements that would not be advisable.

III Supplements (and ergogenic aids) in the spotlight

The one supplement almost everyone is advised to take: vitamin D

Vitamin D is in fact a hormone which regulates calcium and phosphate metabolism. Deficiency of vitamin D causes a medical condition – rickets – in children where there is poor mineralisation of bone. The adult form of vitamin D deficiency is osteomalacia (bone demineralisation). For more information, see Appendix A.

More recently, vitamin D has been shown to have a role in injury risk and recovery, in mental well-being and for the immune system (Cantorna 2010; Wyon et al., 2014; Parker et al., 2017).

There are few foods that contain significant amounts of vitamin D: most of our vitamin D comes from the action of sunlight on skin that starts a process where cholesterol in the body is converted to vitamin D which can then be stored in the liver.

Ballet dancers have been shown to have low levels of vitamin D all year round. In winter levels were lowest and there was a higher incidence of soft tissue injuries (Wolman et al., 2013). Vitamin D supplements in winter have been shown to reduce the incidence of injuries and increase strength in dancers (Wyon et al., 2014). A further study found that before supplementation only 13% of a group of 67 dancers had adequate vitamin D levels before supplementation. The authors concluded that 'vitamin D supplementation decreased the numbers of deficient and insufficient participants within this cohort. The intervention group reported a small significant increase in muscle strength that was negatively associated with traumatic injury occurrence' (Wyon et al., 2018).

The UK currently advises we take 10 micrograms (μg) or 400 international units (i.u.) of vitamin D daily unless we can obtain adequate sunlight. The USA and Europe advise 15 μg or 600 i.u. per day, and not more than 100 μg (4,000 i.u.) daily.

The required dose can be taken either in tablets or via a nasal spray. There is some debate about the overall efficacy of vitamin D supplements, despite the evidence in dancers, but following current advice with regards to supplement dose is advisable. In addition, try and get sunlight exposure: 10–15 minutes daily in between 11 a.m. and 3 p.m. without high-factor sunscreen for vitamin D production (if you are out for longer use a suitable sunscreen for additional time) to benefit from year-round sunshine, which may offer additional health benefits.

The supplements vegans need

For more detail on nutritional challenges of completely plant-based diets see Chapter 12.

Vegans are advised to ensure they have a source of vitamin B12 in their diet, and a dose of at least 1.5 mcg per day is advised. In addition, a source of iodine is advised if you are living in the UK, where salt isn't iodised, or you live where salt is iodised but you use little salt. Most iodine comes from white fish and dairy, so those excluding these foods need a supplement. Currently, only a small number of milk alternatives are supplemented with iodine, if possible use one of these.

The supplements vegetarians and vegans need to think about, relevant to any dancer who avoids fish, meat or dairy products.

Omega-3 fatty acids: these have been discussed in detail in Chapter 6. There is uncertainty over how well humans can use plant-based omega-3 fatty acids. There is evidence that omega-3 fatty acids can reduce inflammation and improve the immune response to tissue damage as well as improve muscle function and blood vessel elasticity. Because of these important benefits to well-being, an omega-3 supplement is advisable. While fish liver oils may be acceptable to some vegetarians, their high vitamin A content makes them far from ideal. Check your supplements to make sure you're not having vitamin A from more than one source (see Appendix A for more information on vitamin A). Look for an omega-3 supplement that provides about 450 mg of EPA and DHA daily. Algal oils are now widely available, and they are the source of omega-3 for fish. Avoid taking more than advised as very high doses (3,000 mg) can prevent necessary blood clotting after injury.

Calcium: including two to three servings from milk, yoghurt, cheese or fortified plant-based alternatives, together with a range of other foods daily will meet your requirements for calcium. If you are not including dairy or fortified alternatives in your nutrition plan, then a supplement would be a good alternative. Look for one that can provide around 700 mg calcium per day. If it is higher, up to 1,500 mg daily and you have few foods rich in calcium there is unlikely to be any problem. Above 1,500 mg supplemental calcium daily may result in digestive issues. High intakes of calcium can interfere with zinc and iron absorption. This is one of many nutrients where an excess over requirements is not beneficial.

The supplements some women may need/find useful

Pre-menopausal women are recommended to take more iron daily than men to account for menstrual losses. Vegetarian and vegan women face an additional challenge as plant sources of iron are less well absorbed than that from meat or fish. Iron availability of vegetarian foods is further reduced by drinking tea or coffee with the meal. Taking this together then a supplement may be needed. If you are feeling unusually tired and blood tests reveal low iron levels then you may be prescribed an iron supplement. These are variably tolerated and can cause nausea, diarrhoea or constipation. If you are unable to tolerate the full dose prescribed the, first option is to ask for an alternative source of iron (e.g., ferrous fumerate rather than ferrous sulphate), or vice versa.

There is some work on the best time to take iron in relation to exercise. The authors of one paper conclude from their research with elite male rowers that it is best to take iron before exercise as exercise increases levels of hepcidin, a hormone which regulates iron absorption, so iron absorption is likely to be lower after exercise (Fensham et al., 2021). It may well also be better to take iron in the morning rather than later in the day (McCormick et al., 2020).

Supplements and ergogenic aids that may have some benefit to some dancers

Questions to ask about ergogenic aids before taking

Question	Consideration
• Is this ergogenic aid safe?	• Check with Informed–Sport or local system.
• Are the benefits of the ergogenic aid based on reliable scientific evidence?	• This requires looking at the product claim(s) and checking the data they cite as evidence.
• How much have I researched about this particular product?	• Check you have enough information to make an informed decision.
• Am I familiar with the brand?	• If the answer is no, then some background checking would be useful.
• Have studies found the product effective in people doing similar levels of activity to me?	• If there are no studies on the brand you are looking at, your best option is to look for a comparable brand with some data.
• Is it potentially a waste of money?	• Check you have clear reasons for taking, and have considered 'food first'.
• Do I think this product is going to make my goals reality?	• Be realistic about how any product can help – it needs to lead significant improvements in performance
• Does this product interact with other supplements or medications?	• Check on any medication you take for any substances that would not be advisable.

A number of widely available supplements are reviewed in Table 8.3. Any dancer wishing to explore using a supplement needs to consider how long it takes before you see any effect, as well as the safety and potential side effects, and accessing from a reliable source. Beta-alanine, for example, needs to be taken for two to four weeks to see any benefit (Trexler et al., 2015). Creatine needs to be taken for at least two weeks to see benefit (Naderi et al., 2016).

The timing of supplements also needs consideration, as this may need to be before exercise, during exercise, after exercise, with meals or before sleep to be effective.

Caffeine

Caffeine is a substance widely used by many dancers, although not always with a focus on achieving enhanced performance (Figure 8.1). While you may not think of caffeine as a supplement, because it occurs naturally in tea, coffee, cocoa and other foods and drinks, it can also be bought as an isolated chemical, as well as being added to some drinks, for example those labelled as 'energy' drinks. From a chemical perspective, caffeine is an alkaloid, a naturally occurring organic nitrogen-containing compound. There are other alkaloids which have wide-ranging and important physiological effects on humans. Well-known alkaloids include morphine, strychnine, quinine, ephedrine and nicotine. The chemical name of caffeine is 1,3,7-trimethylxanthine. In pure form, it is a white powder with a bitter taste that is soluble both in water and fat. Because the structure of caffeine is similar to adenosine, part of ATP (see Chapter 3), it can bind to the receptors of adenosine and this is thought to be the mechanism by which caffeine affects the functioning of the nervous system. Caffeine can increase lipolysis and spare glycogen, stimulate the heart, and cause smooth muscle in the lungs to be more relaxed which may help breathing. All of these may help performance. It can also increase urine output, though research shows that this is unlikely to happen if you are used to drinking up to three to four cups of tea/coffee per day. However, suddenly using high caffeine drinks, or increasing coffee intake significantly, is likely to result in increased urine output which is not helpful for hydration as well as being inconvenient.

Caffeine acts on the nervous system and increases alertness and concentration. It can enhance performance across the range of endurance and high-intensity exercise. Once caffeine is consumed, it is absorbed rapidly, and levels peak in the blood within 45–90 minutes, although it can take as little as 15 minutes or as long as 120 minutes to reach peak levels. Breakdown is slower: the half-life of caffeine (the time it takes to breakdown 50% of a dose of caffeine) is around five hours but can vary between individuals from 1.5 hours up to 9 hours. The differences in breakdown rates are one of the reasons people react differently to caffeine. The rate of caffeine breakdown is influenced by hormones particularly in women, and the oral contraceptive pill (OCP) may slow down caffeine breakdown. For this reason, it's useful to take note of how caffeine works for you.

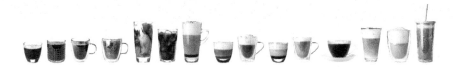

Figure 8.1 Sources of caffeine.
Credit: New Africa/Shutterstock

There is good evidence for the benefits of caffeine; it has been trialled many times in sport. The method of consumption makes little difference (pill, drink). There are side effects in some individuals (increased heart rate, palpitations, anxiety, sleeplessness, etc.). There are recommendations on the dose which can be useful to enhance performance without resulting in unwanted side effects.

Considerations for caffeine use

The dose: typically 1–3 mg per kg body weight is used for strength and endurance activities, taken fairly close to exercise starting. This is a good starting dose if you want to compare your intake to doses used to enhance performance. Typically 5–9 mg per kg body weight are considered high doses. Typically 3–6 mg per kg body weight is a range that is likely to improve performance but not cause side effects such as sleeplessness and anxiety. Using drinks as your source of caffeine is less precise than using a measured dose from a caffeine product, and depending on the dose you are aiming for could be a significant volume to drink, but is a more familiar option than manufactured gels, gums, tablets or shots.

Timing: if you are thinking about how caffeine can best support training or performance then timing is important. Allowing about an hour from taking caffeine to when you want the most effect is a good starting point and you can then experiment to see if your individual metabolism makes it more effective to have the caffeine sooner or later than this.

Your liver breaks down caffeine. About 85% is converted into paraxanthine, 10% to theobromine and 15% to theophylline, all of which have physiological effects. Paraxanthine may contribute to development of tolerance and withdrawal symptoms if caffeine is taken regularly.

Caffeine in a mouth rinse may also be effective in the very short term, such as for a very short intense piece of a dance performance – it has been shown to be effective for cyclists for sprints, although overall the evidence is mixed so far in sport (Ehlert et al., 2020). As always, if you want to see if this could help your performance make sure you first test it out in a class or rehearsal where it is less of a problem if you the effect is not as you expect.

The recommended upper intake of caffeine per day is 200 mg in one drink and 400 mg in total daily. Table 8.2 shows the caffeine content of a number of caffeine-containing drinks.

Creatine

Creatine is a natural compound found in the body. Typically, an omnivorous diet will provide 1–2 g creatine per day from meat and fish, which results in muscle stores being about 60–80% saturated. Creatine is made of three amino acids: arginine, glycine and methionine. Its effect on performance is seen when it combines with phosphorus to make phosphocreatine (PCr) in muscle cells. There is normally only enough creatine in the body to

Table 8.2 Caffeine content of drinks

Drink	Amount (ml)	Approx caffeine content (mg)
Tea, black cup/small mug	225	50
Filter coffee cup/small mug	225	95
Instant coffee cup/small mug	225	60+ (higher if stronger)
Single Espresso shot	45	65–100
Energy drink large can	500	160
Hot chocolate cup/small mug	225	<10
Cola	330	35–40
Diet cola	330	42
Green tea	225	30

Data based on European Food Safety Authority, research data and manufacturers' information.

fuel around 10 seconds of high-intensity activity. Supplements can increase natural levels by about 30%. Research has indicated that as well as improving performance by enhanced acute exercise capacity and training adaptations, creatine supplementation may increase lean body mass, enhance post-exercise recovery, injury prevention, thermoregulation, rehabilitation and concussion and/or spinal cord neuroprotection.

There have been many studies looked into the benefits of creatine. Creatine monohydrate is the form of creatine most studied. Research shows that it is most useful for high-intensity short-term activities, for example, lifting weights and for explosive actions such as jumps. It has been shown to be safe both in the short and long terms. Supplementation up to 30 g per day for five years is safe and well-tolerated in healthy individuals, and possibly health benefits from taking 3 g per day long term (Kreider et al., 2017). One disadvantage is that in some people taking creatine can lead to 1–3 kg weight gain due to extra water being held in muscle. Any increased muscle mass will also increase body weight, but this also brings potential benefits, which water retention doesn't.

Historically, there has been a loading dose phase, up to 20 g per day, spread over at least four doses, for a period of 5–7 days followed by a maintenance dose longer term of 3–5 g per day as a single daily dose. Missing out the loading phase is a more recent option that will also increase stores of creatine in muscle, though over a slightly longer time period than a week. Taking with carbohydrate alone, or carbohydrate and protein, promotes greater creatine retention in the body.

Dancers considering taking creatine need to weigh up the possible advantages of improved performance with the potential disadvantage of having additional weight to lift when jumping if water retention does occur. Always optimise your diet before looking at performance enhancing supplements to get the most consistent benefits.

Carbohydrate supplements

Carbohydrate supplements are widely used by endurance athletes to maintain energy levels over long events in a form that is well tolerated by the body. Research has been done to find the amounts and types of carbohydrate that can be tolerated hourly when undertaking long events, typically running or cycling (Reynolds et al., 2022). Carbohydrate gels are easily available for these situations and provide around 22 g carbohydrate per portion with a recommendation from manufacturers to take up to 3 sachets, 66 g carb per hour, which is at the upper end of the recommendation for 30–60 g per hour for exercise up to 2.5 hours duration. It is also the maximum many dancers will tolerate without practice taking and ensuring that combinations of different types of carbohydrate are used. The carbohydrate in gels is typically from maltodextrin (carbohydrate derived from corn starch, consisting of 4–20 glucose units) or maltodextrin with glucose and/or fructose. Many also contain some electrolytes, usually sodium and potassium. Some also contain caffeine. Carbohydrate supplements have been shown to delay fatigue and increase endurance. Adequate fluids are needed alongside the gels, although many can be taken alone as long as overall fluid intake is regular and adequate.

'Energy' drinks usually provide around 10–12 g carbohydrate per 100 ml (unless they are a low sugar drink with a high dose of caffeine), but in a much larger volume. As a supplement for performance, high carbohydrate energy drinks are often not an ideal option for dancers as the fluid is slow to be absorbed, which may impair performance. Typically, you would need around 200 ml of an energy drink to get 20–25 g carbohydrate. An isotonic sports drink would be a better option as it would provide around 10–14 g carb in 200 ml, with some electrolytes, and the fluid would be absorbed relatively fast, helping you stay hydrated while also giving a useful amount of carbs. For best nutrient intake, getting carbs mostly from food is advisable, using a supplement only when food intake is limited.

Protein supplements

Protein supplements may be from milk (whey or casein), egg or can be plant based such as from pea, rice or hemp protein. They are sold as powders, though there are also high protein products such as bars or drinks available to buy which are often more expensive compared with a basic powder protein source. Protein powders usually provide 20–25 g protein per scoop, and the bars and drinks provide up to this amount. If you struggle to eat protein-rich foods or to eat the amounts recommended, which is not uncommon, then a protein supplement can be a useful way to make up the difference between the amount you can typically manage to eat on average and your target intake. There is no major disadvantage to using a protein supplement, though a minor disadvantage is that you won't generally be getting the other nutrients that go along with protein in food.

If you are using a plant-based protein, then if possible check the leucine content as this is known to be important for muscle protein synthesis – more on this in Chapter 5.

Electrolytes

Food is a great source of the electrolytes you need, and providing you are able to eat regularly you may well be able to meet all your electrolyte requirements under most circumstances. Potassium is found in many foods, particularly fruits, vegetables and salads, so including 5+ portions a day will provide a good intake. Sodium as sodium chloride is every day table or cooking salt, used in many foods, and often added in cooking and/or at the table. Excess sodium chloride is not advisable for general health. Magnesium is the third electrolyte typically used in electrolyte supplements. Magnesium is found in a range of foods, see Appendix A. As magnesium can cause gut disturbances in excess, make sure to follow the guidelines for making up and maximum daily intakes if you do use electrolyte supplements. Sometimes a small amount of calcium is also added, which is a fraction of the amount you will obtain from food.

Electrolyte supplements may be useful for situations when sweat losses are high, for example, if you are dancing in a hot climate without air conditioning, or you naturally have a higher rate of sweat loss than others, or lose more salt in sweat – one indication is if you notice more white marks than others when sweat dries on dark clothing. If you need to drink over 4 l per day then again an electrolyte supplement is worth trialling.

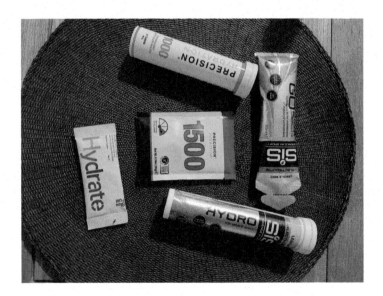

Photo 8.2 Electrolyte supplements.

Electrolytes may also be worth trialling if you have a high dance work-load and normally use mostly home-prepared food, use very little salt in cooking and don't include high salt foods such as cheese, ham, bacon, sausages (meat or vegan/vegetarian) in your normal diet. As always if you decide to trial something new, pick a time when it will matter less if you get any unexpected effects (unlikely with electrolytes taken as advised by reputable manufacturers). Some products use sorbitol as a sweetener which can cause gut issues in excess. Also, it's always best to only trial one new nutrition strategy at a time, when the rest of your schedule is fairly stable, so you can accurately assess how well the new strategy works for you.

Probiotics

A quick reminder that probiotics are products containing live micro-organisms that are known to be helpful to human health and are found naturally in the gut. Probiotic supplements can be drinks/yoghurt products, or in the form of pills or capsules. Price varies hugely; one reason being that some products have been well researched which adds to costs. From a performance perspective probiotics don't have a direct impact but can support health, gastrointestinal function and immunity.

Taking a probiotic supplement at the beginning of a course of antibiotics and for at least a week can reduce the risks of the antibiotic causing gut disturbances.

Travel abroad can increase the risk of gut problems such as diarrhoea. Taking a probiotic containing *Saccharomyces boulardii* or a probiotics product containing *Lactobacillus acidophilus* and *Bifidobacterium bifidum* during the trip help you avoid gut problems.

Finally, if you suffer from constipation and have made changes to increase your fibre intake and your fluid intake is adequate, then a four-week trial of a probiotic containing Bifidobacterium lactis is worth considering. Those with IBS may benefit from a probiotic specifically formulated to help with this. Again a four-week trial initially is the best way to start.

And which supplements aren't worth the money/aren't effective/could be harmful?

There are many supplements which either aren't effective – they don't actually give the benefits they claim, or actually can cause harm. For others, no benefits have yet been shown though this may change over time. There isn't enough space in this chapter to cover all of these, so if you are interested in other supplements your best strategy is a literature search to see the current evidence.

Some supplements currently in the 'lack of evidence' category, and which dancers are not advised to take, are β-hydroxy-β-methylbutyrate (HMB), seaweed extract fucoxanthin, co-enzyme Q10, chromium and bee pollen. Others, such as ketone bodies, are extremely expensive and unpalatable, so not advisable until and unless there is clear evidence of any benefit. Another group can be harmful; a number of these are included in Table 8.3.

NB in the table above the term 'performance' means the ability to perform physical work, e.g., complete dance sequences with precision and danced full out. Products are categorised as supplements and/or ergogenic aids depending on whether they can benefit health, performance, or both.

Table 8.3 A summary of supplements and ergogenic aids

Product S = Supplement Erg A = Ergogenic aid	What are the claims?	What does it contain that might be useful?	How good is the evidence?	Is it useful for dancers?
Amino acids (single) S, Erg A	Enhance responses to training and improve recovery	Specified amino acids	Difficult to assess as effects will depend on how adequate diet is. Leucine known to be beneficial for stimulating muscle protein synthesis	Possibly under specific circumstances, get specialist advice. Improving total protein intake best strategy particularly considering leucine intake
Antioxidants S/Erg A	Reduce fatigue by reducing damage to cells from free radicals	Beta-carotene Vitamin C, vitamin E	No clear benefit, and supplements may reduce recovery	Only likely to be useful in deficiency. Focus on adequate intake from food
Beetroot juice: shots of around 70 ml Erg A	Improving performance, increase in stamina	Nitrate: which can be converted into nitric acid in the body	Good evidence for impact on performance in endurance and high-intensity activities	Potentially yes, work on optimising diet first. Long-term use needs research and may not be advisable

(Continued)

Table 8.3 (Continued)

Product S = Supplement Erg A = Ergogenic aid	What are the claims?	What does it contain that might be useful?	How good is the evidence?	Is it useful for dancers?
Beta-alanine Erg A	Increases muscle's ability to tolerate high-intensity exercise for longer (1–4 minutes)	The amino acid beta-alanine, needed to make carnosine (carnosine is histidine and beta-alanine)	Carnosine is an important pH buffer found naturally in muscles. Small studies in sport suggest increased levels from a supplement of beta-alanine may have a small benefit on sustained, high-intensity exercise. Likely to need to take for several weeks to see any effect	Further research required, especially in dance. Long-term effects are not known. Risk of tingling in fingers which may be unhelpful for performance.
Bicarbonate Erg A	Improvement in high-intensity events 1–7 minutes in duration	Sodium bicarbonate is a pH buffer that helps maintain pH in cells and blood	2% performance enhancement	Significant risk of side effects (gastrointestinal upset, nausea, diarrhoea, water retention) so trial with caution if at all
Branch Chain Amino Acids (BCAA) Erg A	Stimulate muscle protein synthesis	BCAA, most likely that leucine is the BCAA that is effective	Some for BCAA, better for leucine	Work on protein intake, consider sources of leucine rather than BCAA, only use tested source if supplement considered
Cannabidiol (CBD) Erg A	Improved sleep, reduced pain, anti-oxidant, anti-inflammatory, helps with anxiety	Cannabinoids	Not yet good enough to suggest dancers should trial or use	Unknown as yet
Carbohydrate gel/drink S/Erg A	Improve performance when carbohydrate stores are limited	Rapidly absorbed carbohydrate	Good evidence	Best to work on meeting requirements, possibly useful in high energy demand times

Product S = Supplement Erg A = Ergogenic aid	What are the claims?	What does it contain that might be useful?	How good is the evidence?	Is it useful for dancers?
L-Carnitine Erg A	Enhanced exercise capacity and endurance	L-Carnitine, important role in fatty acid oxidation in the liver and heart. Synthesised from essential amino acids lysine and methionine	Good evidence, generally positive, though not always showing benefits	Optimise diet before considering use. Research details including side effects and risks before taking.
Casein S/Erg A	Increase muscle accretion when taken after resistance exercise	Amino acids including leucine: slower to digest than whey protein, effects can be less	Good quality though most research focuses on whey protein. Mixed reports whey versus casein.	Useful if looking for muscle gain and undertaking resistance exercise: whey may be the better option
Collagen Erg A	Promote joint health and support injury recovery	Collagen	Lack of evidence in elite performers, though some evidence in other groups	Thought to be safe, optimise diet first, before considering using
Gelatin Erg A	Improve collagen synthesis	Amino acids similar profile to collagen	Small studies with vitamin C and gelatin	Focus on adequate protein and vitamin C before considering gelatin
Ginger (Zingiber officinale) S/Erg A	Increase metabolic rate and isometric force generation. Reduce the inflammatory response to exercise.	Active elements not clear	Few studies, lack of evidence	Not yet enough evidence to recommend
Ginseng Erg A	Improve performance	Ginsenosides	Lack of evidence as often combined with caffeine and glucose	Better to focus on overall diet and possibly a supplement shown to be effective and safe

(Continued)

Table 8.3 (Continued)

Product S = Supplement Erg A = Ergogenic aid	What are the claims?	What does it contain that might be useful?	How good is the evidence?	Is it useful for dancers?
Glucosamine Erg A	Protects against osteoarthritis	Glucosamine, can be used to synthesise proteoglycans needed for cartilage	Some data that it is effective in adults who have osteoarthritis, data is not consistent though	Lack of data for a protective effect. Only worth considering for those with osteoarthritis currently
Green tea Erg A	Delay fatigue in prolonged exercise	Flavonoids	Mixed data on efficacy	Not yet enough evidence to recommend
Peppermint mouth rinse 0.01–0.1% menthol solution Erg A	Cooling effect to improve heat tolerance	Menthol	Limited but encouraging	Consider if needing to dance in very hot environments
Plant sterols Erg A	Reduce the negative effect of exercise on the immune system	Specific plant sterols, e.g., sitosterol	Limited	Better to focus on including a good range of plant- based foods
Pomegranate Juice Erg A	Recovery from muscle damage	Phytochemicals	Good	Worth considering especially if diet is already varied and well-balanced
Turmeric/ curcumin Erg A	Anti- inflammatory	Curcumin	Benefits to recovery or performance are yet to be clearly demonstrated	Lack of data as yet, best to focus on including a wide range of plant-based foods
Vitamin C S/Erg A	Promote collagen synthesis in joints	Vitamin C	Lack of data currently	Not recommended, though good intake of fruit and vegetables advisable
Whey protein S/Erg A	Increase muscle accretion when taken after resistance exercise	Amino acids including leucine	Good quality	Useful if looking for muscle gain and undertaking resistance exercise

Product S = Supplement Erg A = Ergogenic aid	What are the claims?	What does it contain that might be useful?	How good is the evidence?	Is it useful for dancers?
Yerba Mate (can be used as a tea, or an ingredient in supplements) Erg A	Can help health and performance	A number of compounds including caffeine and phytochemicals, vitamins and minerals	Good evidence for caffeine, little for Yerba mate and may cause side effects	Not recommended
Yohimbine – tree extract from W Africa Erg A	Enhance endurance	Yohimbine	No evidence	Not advised
Yucca extracts Erg A	Can help health and possibly performance	Yuccaols, resveratrol and saponins	No evidence	Not recommended

IV Resources

BMJ/BJSM A–Z of nutritional supplements: dietary supplements, sports nutrition foods and ergogenic aids for health and performance.

Bongiovanni, T., Genovesi, F., Nemmer, M., Carling, C., Alberti, G., How-atson, G. (2020). Nutritional interventions for reducing the signs and symptoms of exercise-induced muscle damage and accelerate recovery in athletes: Current knowledge, practical application and future perspectives. *European Journal of Applied Physiology*, 120(9), pp. 1965–1996.

V Learning outcomes

After reading this chapter the dancer should be able to:

1   Explain the difference between supplements and ergogenic aids.
2   Give three examples of supplements some dancers might need.
3   Discuss the advantages and disadvantages of caffeine for dancers.
4   State potential risks of using supplements that are not batch tested.

References

Cantorna, M.T. (2010) Mechanisms underlying the effect of vitamin D on the im-mune system, *Proceedings of the Nutrition Society*, 69(3), pp.286–289.

Ehlert, A.M., Twiddy, H.M. and Wilson, P.B. (2020) The effects of caffeine mouth rinsing on exercise performance: A systematic review, *International Journal of Sport Nutrition and Exercise Metabolism*, 30(5), pp.362–373.

Fensham, N.C. et al. (2021a) Sequential submaximal training in elite male rowers does not result in amplified increases in interleukin-6 or hepcidin, *International Journal of Sport Nutrition and Exercise Metabolism*, 1(aop), pp.1–9.

Fensham, N.C. et al. (2021b) Sequential submaximal training in elite male rowers does not result in amplified increases in interleukin-6 or hepcidin, *International Journal of Sport Nutrition and Exercise Metabolism*, 1(aop), pp.1–9.

Kreider, R.B. et al. (2017) International society of sports nutrition position stand: Safety and efficacy of creatine supplementation in exercise, sport, and medicine, *Journal of the International Society of Sports Nutrition*, 14(1), pp.1–18.

Maughan, R.J. et al. (2018) IOC consensus statement: Dietary supplements and the high-performance athlete, *International Journal of Sport Nutrition and Exercise Metabolism*, 28(2), pp.104–125.

McCormick, R. et al. (2020) Refining treatment strategies for iron deficient athletes, *Sports Medicine*, 50(12), pp.2111–2123.

Naderi, A. et al. (2016) Timing, optimal dose and intake duration of dietary supplements with evidence-based use in sports nutrition, *Journal of Exercise Nutrition & Biochemistry*, 20(4), p.1.

Parker, G.B., Brotchie, H. and Graham, R.K. (2017) Vitamin D and depression, *Journal of Affective Disorders*, 208, pp.56–61.

Reynolds, K.M. et al. (2022) A food first approach to carbohydrate supplementation in endurance exercise: A systematic review, *International Journal of Sport Nutrition and Exercise Metabolism*, 1(aop), pp.1–15.

Thein, L.A., Thein, J.M. and Landry, G.L. (1995) Ergogenic aids, *Physical Therapy*, 75(5), pp.426–439.

Trexler, E.T. et al. (2015) International society of sports nutrition position stand: Beta-alanine, *Journal of the International Society of Sports Nutrition*, 12(1), pp.1–14.

Wolman, R. et al. (2013) Vitamin D status in professional ballet dancers: Winter vs. summer, *Journal of Science and Medicine in Sport*, 16(5), pp.388–391.

Wyon, M.A. et al. (2014) The influence of winter vitamin D supplementation on muscle function and injury occurrence in elite ballet dancers: A controlled study, *Journal of Science and Medicine in Sport*, 17(1), pp.8–12.

Wyon, M.A. et al. (2018) The effect of vitamin D supplementation in elite adolescent dancers on muscle function and injury incidence: A randomised double-blind study, *International Journal of Sports Physiology and Performance*, pp.1–15.

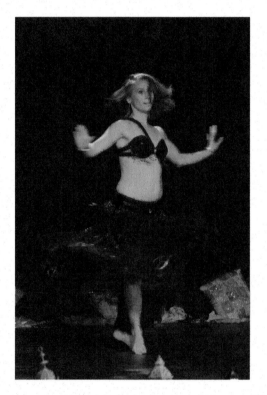

Photo 9.1 Dynamic movement comes from the co-ordination of the amazing structures that are connected together to make a dancer's body.
Photo courtesy of Steve Scadden.

9 Body composition

Contents

I The dancer's physique: the many components of fitness

Currently a significant proportion of dancers probably experience more comments about their physique than in almost any other area of life, second only to technique corrections/feedback. Physique can be defined as 'the form, size, and development of a person's body', or, more simply, as the shape and size of your body.

It used to be common practice for some critics reviewing ballets to include comments, sometimes very negative, on dancers' physiques, without this necessarily being related to their dancing. This is now generally seen as both unnecessary, and unacceptable. To be clear: there is a world of difference between criticising a dance performance, which is the subjective view of the person who has watched the performance, and insulting a dancer's body, when it has nothing to do with the performance and is neither useful nor acceptable and may potentially cause distress and harm to that dancer. There has been recent discussion in the media about 'ballet bodies', which raises a host of issues:

1   Is there a particular body shape and size that can do ballet, and other bodies cannot do ballet?
2   How does body shape relate to ability to dance?

DOI: 10.4324/9781003219002-9

3   Looking on social media you can find clips of many shapes and sizes performing and enjoying ballet, so who is defining the criteria of what a 'ballet body' should look like?

4   If a dancer has to severely restrict their nutritional intake to achieve what someone who has power over them requires of their body, is this a healthy situation for the world of dance? Of course, it is not healthy for the dancer.

Ballet is the dance form where there is most controversy over physique, and the most pressure to conform to a particular look, hence the focus on this dance genre. But it is not exclusive to ballet.

Physique can and does change over time. Initially, through growth and maturation from a child's body into an adult body there are many changes which take place in terms not just of height, but of proportions, muscle and body fat content and frame shape. Growth can continue much longer than is often considered. Although men typically finish gaining height by the age of 18, some can still be gaining height up to the age of 21, or even older if their adolescent growth spurt was delayed – which it can be by inadequate nutrition and/or high training load. Women may have finished growing by the age of 16 but can continue gaining height until the age of 18 years.

Once men have achieved their full height, there are still changes in body shape that need to occur, in particular chest depth, which increases. For women, once adult height is reached, the pelvic area continues to increase to reach a maximum in early adulthood (Berger et al., 2011). It may then reduce slightly (Huseynov et al., 2016).

Ideally, you have been able to have access to a wide range of foods and have had a healthy relationship with food, where you use it to meet your requirements and seen it as – hopefully – enjoyable fuel with a social role. Your body will have grown and developed through childhood and adolescence and by adulthood you find yourself with a body that is strong enough, flexible enough and with enough stamina to undertake the dance you love in a way that you can enjoy. Your physique is unique to you, nobody is perfect, we are humans and the human body has vulnerabilities.

In sport, there has long been a focus on achieving a body that is optimal for the sport. The question is how does this apply to dance? To start it's helpful to take a moment to clarify the various aspects of the human body in exercise that are often regarded as parts of fitness. Keeping it simple there are three main components:

Cardiovascular endurance (aerobic power) and muscular endurance – often summarised as stamina
Strength and power/explosive strength
Flexibility

Agility, balance and co-ordination may be included but to some extent are dependent on strength and flexibility. Reaction time and speed are sometimes included but again will depend on having sufficient strength and power to optimise these. Body composition is also sometimes included as a component of fitness; this will be explored further through this chapter.

There can be some trade-offs when looking at improving the main components of fitness. It is now accepted that increasing strength without developing large muscles is perfectly possible and also that increasing muscle size does not necessarily impact on flexibility, if appropriate stretching regimes are undertaken. But focussing on flexibility and neglecting to work on strength is unhelpful for dancers. Stamina is often overlooked but is crucial to be able to complete rehearsals and performances. Athletes from different disciplines can look very different: just picture a high jumper for a moment, and then a shot putter: they need to have very different physiques to perform effectively. High jumpers benefit from being taller and are often lean as it is potentially easier to propel their weight upwards if body fat is lower rather than higher. But muscle strength is crucial, and a low body weight with no consideration of body composition is not a successful formula. Chapter 11 discusses the need for an adequate, healthy level of body fat for the body to function effectively. Shot putters need strength and power to propel the shot forwards, and research suggests that body composition is not related to performance (Terzis et al., 2012). Dancers are more similar to those participating in many team sports as they use a wider range of movements compared with many single athletic disciplines, and the focus should be on a body that is fit for purpose, remembering that body composition on its own is not necessarily any indicator of success in performance. There is a myth that dancers have to be light for a partner to lift them. While there are safety considerations for sure if a dancer is going to lift another dancer who is at much higher weight, the techniques of both dancers are crucial. A dancer at low weight, who is not well nourished, who is not strong, and who has limited energy due to inadequate nutrition is likely to be harder to lift than a fit and healthy dancer who may be several kilos heavier but plays a more active part in the lift. Unfortunately, if the low-weight dancer perceives they are not as easy to lift as another dancer they may interpret this as meaning they need to be lighter still. There is a difference in the age that male and female dancers reach full maturity, with males reaching this on average at least one year later. This difference means teachers have a challenge matching males and females for partner work to ensure the right levels of skills and strength.

II Nutrition and the adolescent pubertal period

There are many changes that the dancer's body go through between the ages of around 10–24 years of age (Sawyer et al., 2018). Growth is complex: different body tissues in the same body part may grow at different rates, so bones, muscles, tendons and ligaments are not all growing at the same rate. But also, different body parts grow at different times: feet grow before lower legs/arms, then upper legs/arms while the final section to grow is the trunk. And while all this is going on there are changing hormone levels, and development of the mature adult body, which for females involves breast development. Centre of gravity changes, movement can become harder as muscle strength takes a while to catch up after growth and all of this can be stressful for the young dancer who can feel as if they are not making the progress they expect with their training. Peak rate of height gain in biological females occurs roughly between 6 and 12 months before menstrual periods start and peak weight spurt. Males typically have more height to gain, and this starts at a slightly later age, with the weight spurt starting at about the same time as the height spurt.

From the start of the adolescent growth spurt nutrient requirements for males and females start to diverge, as males gradually gain both height and muscle volume compared with females. From the time menstrual periods start for females, there is an increased requirement for iron, which it is helpful to be aware of, particularly as those whose intake is mostly plant based may benefit from guidance on iron-rich foods. See Appendix A. Once periods start for females the next stage of growth is one of body fat levels moving to a more adult level. This can be difficult for the earlier developers, who may feel that they are 'bigger' than their peers: which may indeed be the case, but not because they are too big. This is a stage where dance teachers can be supportive to young dancers, and there is research exploring this (Mitchell et al., 2017). Initially, girls can be taller than boys the same age, but over the next few years, everyone reaches their adult height and mature body. Time is required to see the height and proportions of every young dancer's adult body. There is additional research looking at the risks of talented dancers leaving dance after puberty because they feel that they no longer look appropriate for dance (Mitchell et al., 2016).

III Body composition

Your body is unique, yet the variation between your body and that of other dancers may be less than you think. Although data from analysis of dancers' body composition is limited, it can still useful to be aware of some elements of body composition.

Water

Typically adults are around 60% water. This water is present in every cell of the human body and, in fact, makes up a significant amount of many cells. Muscle is around 75% water, and our blood volume – around 4 l for female dancers and 5 l for male dancers – is over 60% percent water. All the organs of the body have a high water content. Even body fat, which has a crucial role insulating and protecting the body, contains at least 15% water. Dehydration has a potential impact on the whole body, and indeed a 2% loss of body weight from dehydration has an impact on your ability to perform movement to your normal standard.

The actual percentage of water in your body is constantly changing. You take in water in food and drinks, digest and absorb it, lose fluid through sweat, breath, and from the gut and in urine. Homeostasis is the term used where your body is able to regulate the amount of not just water but also mineral salts to help keep your body functioning at its best. Thirst is the mechanism which drives homeostasis and aims to ensure your fluid intake replaces losses. Hydration is looked at in Chapter 7.

Protein

From the perspective of body composition, it is useful to remember that protein is found in muscle, as well as in tendons, ligaments, cartilage, bone, skin, hair, nails, blood cells and even in fat cells.

Minerals

Your body contains around 1kg of calcium, plus smaller amounts of a range of other minerals such as sodium, potassium, phosphorous, chlorine, magnesium, manganese, zinc and iodine which are all needed for a huge number of roles in health and performance. For details of minerals needed by the body, see Appendix A.

Fat

Fat within the human body has a number of vital functions. Firstly, it is there as an energy source. This is a major role, but there are a number of others which will be reviewed. Healthy levels of body fat act as the biggest reserve of energy a dancer has. The store of carbohydrate by comparison is extremely small, and so needs regular replenishment. If carbohydrate reserves are adequate, and through regular meals and snacks are regularly replaced, and you have healthy levels of body fat, then all levels of dance activity can be fuelled – and at most levels of exercise intensity fats can be used together with carbs. The proportion of fat used as fuel reduces as the level of dance intensity increases. For high-intensity activity, then carbs are the fuel required. If carb stores run out in the working muscles and blood sugar levels drop, you will struggle to keep dancing at the intensity required until more carbs are ingested. Fat becomes the only realistic fuel option; the body is designed to do this – fat use increases when insulin levels are low, which is when blood glucose levels are low. Using fat as the main fuel though does mean having to work at lower intensity, which obviously limits dance options.

Lipolysis is the process describing the release of fatty acids from reserve fat stores in the body. The opposite process, lipogenesis, is where fat can be stored when the body has a high fat and/or carbohydrate intake. Your body regulates the processes carefully to manage energy stores and energy availability in your body. Exercise increases lipolysis at lower intensity exercise, when fat can be used as a fuel, but at higher intensities lipolysis does not increase. Stress can also increase lipolysis.

Additional roles for fat in the body

- Insulation
- Protection of internal organs
- Production of hormones
- Protection of bones, for example the backside – too little fat on your backside can make it uncomfortable to sit
- Fat is an essential component of cell membranes throughout the body
- As the main building block for steroid hormones such as oestrogen and testosterone as well as cortisol produced by the adrenal glands

There is an amount of body fat referred to as 'essential fat' which is needed for insulation, protecting vital organs, for vitamin storage, and production of hormones. Essential body fat is approximately 3% of body mass for men and 12% of body mass for women. In addition to this, there is an amount of storage fat, which is also essential for the body to function properly. Healthy levels of body fat are regarded as around 17–25% for young women, increasing slightly with age. Some female dancers may naturally have slightly lower levels and still be healthy, but this will not be typical. Healthy levels of body fat for men are 13–20%, though some male dancers can be healthy with natural body fat levels below 10%.

Body composition myths and facts

Myth	Fact	Note
Tracking weight changes is a good way to track changes in body fat and/or muscle content	Your body is about 60% water, but this varies mainly due to intake and activity so most weight fluctuations are water not muscle or fat	Weighing can cause significant stress and is of limited value for most adult dancers
There is a perfect weight for height for dancers	Weight takes no account of body composition or frame	Reported heights and weights of other dancers and tables of 'dancer' heights and weights are not useful
Dancers need to be as light as possible for partners to lift them	Strength and technique are important for successful lifts: a dancer who weighs more but uses good technique is easier to lift than a lighter dancer who doesn't	Being below your healthy weight range increases the risk of injuries both short and long term
Eating more protein leads to muscle gain	Increases in muscle strength and size only happen if there is enough protein and energy and a physical workload designed to build muscle	Dancers need more protein than sedentary people: this can be a challenge particularly for vegetarian or vegan dancers – see Chapter 5

Body composition models

Measuring body composition in sport has been a regular procedure for many years. This can be for several reasons. For those in weight category sports, where often participants will be competing at weighs below their natural healthy weight, the aim will be to maintain muscle mass while reducing fat mass, with the aim of optimising strength and power. For other sports, it can be to check that athletes have a good level of muscle rather than lower muscle higher fat levels, again with the aim of optimising performance. Knowing roughly the amount of muscle mass or body fat in a dancer's body may be interesting to the dancer and dance scientists, who can use the information to potentially see if there are levels of body composition that allow dancers perhaps to reduce their risk of injuries, or to achieve measurable levels of skills such as jump height, as performance is less easily measured in dance.

Looking at the ways of separating the body into different components, there are currently three main models. The original model was a two-compartment model, which separated the body into fat-free mass, which includes muscle, bone, organs, connective tissues and water, and fat mass. The three-compartment model separates out bone from the remainder of the fat-free mass. The four-compartment model estimates amounts of water, protein mass, and bone and fat. Multicompartment models sub-divide lean mass components further. Table 9.1 shows the details of the various models used for considering body composition.

The more compartments that are used the more detail you have about the composition of your body. The compartment of most interest and relevance is that of fat-free mass, as this is the information that is useful for exploring whether a dancer has low or adequate energy availability.

Assessing body composition

Knowing a dancer's height and weight tells us nothing about their body composition. Calculating body mass index, which is weight (kg) divided by

Table 9.1 Body composition models

One-compartment model	Two-compartment model	Three-compartment model	Four-compartment model	Multicompartment model
Weight				Essential fat
	Fat mass	Fat mass	Fat mass	Storage fat
	Fat-free mass	Fat-free mass	Total body water	Total body water
		Bone	Lean mass	Protein
			Bone mineral	Bone mineral
				Soft tissue mineral
				Glycogen

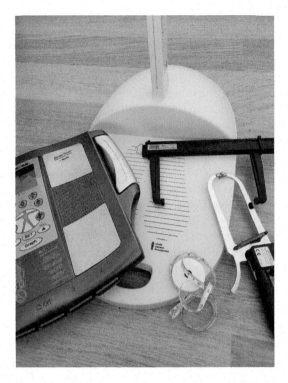

Photo 9.2 Accuracy of body composition measurement depends on the equipment and the skills of those using it.

height in metre square, has some value to identify health risks at very low (adult BMI under 17) and very high (adult BMI over 35) values but otherwise gives no information as to whether body fat levels or muscle mass levels are at levels which will support good health and performance.

Some dancers have no interest in the exact details of their body composition, although they are likely to be very invested in having a body that has strong enough bones, adequate body fat and suitable amounts of muscles as well as healthy organs. Other dancers may be keen to know what the proportions of muscle and fat are in their body. If this is coming from a place of acceptance of their body, rather than critical thoughts, with an interest as to how body composition might impact on aspects of dance technique, then undertaking body composition assessment, perhaps as part of a study, or to compare against research data, is not unreasonable. The challenge is to find techniques which are accessible and give meaningful accuracy.

The gold standard technique for measuring body composition is MRI scanning, which historically has been both expensive and time to consuming to analyse. This will likely improve over time, and may become accessible but is currently really only a research tool.

DEXA (dual energy X-ray absorptiometry) which uses a very low dose of X-rays to produce a scan of the body and interpretations of what the scan means, is not widely available for whole body composition measurement, but is more available than MRI.

The BOD POD works by measuring the amount of air you displace inside a closed container – the technical description for this technique is air displacement plethysmography. Specific formulae are applied to the result to produce body composition data. This is a two-compartment model so doesn't give as much information as a three- or four-compartment model would. Nonetheless, the BOD POD is a reliable technique and BOD PODS is more widely accessible than DEXA or MRI scanners for body composition.

Underwater weighing is a similar technique to the BOD POD, where the weight underwater is compared to the weight in air. The difference of the body weight in air and water is used to calculate the body's density. From this density formulae previously derived are used to predict the amounts of fat-free mass and fat mass in the body. This is one of the first techniques that were available, and for many years it was the gold standard technique. It is again a two-compartment model. The equipment is relatively inexpensive, requiring a large tank of water and a means to weigh an individual underwater, for example, a chair in the tank that is attached to weighing scales. The challenge to the participant is that the lungs need to be as empty as possible in the underwater weighing, and holding your breath with empty lungs while the scale steadies is considerably harder than with full lungs.

A widely accessible technology for measuring body composition is bioelectrical impedance analysis (BIA). BIA estimates body fat percentage by measuring the resistance of a very small amount of electrical current flowing through the body. Different types of body tissue resist electricity in different ways; muscle is a good conductor and fat is a poor conductor of electric current. The equipment then uses equations derived from research to translate the amount of current which passes through the body into an estimate of body composition. BIA equipment may require users to stand on a set of scales with electrodes embedded which runs a very small amount of electrical current through just the feet, while other more sophisticated equipment requires current to run through both arms and legs. More sophisticated equipment has increased accuracy and reliability. Readings are affected by exercise, eating and drinking, and will not be valid if the required conditions for measuring are not met.

Research has shown that while BIA scales are widely available and give very precise results, often to one or two decimal places, unfortunately the accuracy of these precise numbers is limited, and may be several kilo's out in estimating lean and fat mass (Borga et al., 2018). There are more complex versions of this technology which give more accurate data, with the potential advantage of separating intra-cellular water (ICW) from extra-cellular water

(ECW). There are some data on the differences in the ratios between athletes and more sedentary people but as yet no clear use of this information in either sport or dance.

A final technique that many dancers will have come across is the use of skinfold callipers. These are relatively inexpensive, but for best results, it is essential to use one of the small number of brands which are recognised as sufficiently accurate. The callipers are used to identify the thickness of a fold of skin, with the underlying layer of fat, on a number of sites of the body to reach a total for the selected number of sites. Measurements should only be undertaken by those who have undertaken training, as the measurement sites are precisely located, and there are specific techniques for taking the measurement. Even so there is a small degree of error, minimised if repeated measurements over time are carried out by the same person. While the total of the skinfold measurements can be compared to tables where equations have been used which translate skinfold thicknesses to body fat percentages, this introduces further errors as the equations have been derived from groups who may not be representative of dancer bodies. One potential use of skinfold measurements is to see whether changes in skinfold thicknesses over time in healthy dancers correlate with injury frequencies or changes in specific aspects of dance technique. Another option would be the comparison of groups of dancers again to identify norms for specific genres or techniques, or injury rates that may be linked to body composition.

Dancers with disabilities

Studies on body composition have been undertaken in paralympic athletes to assess whether there are characteristics of more successful athletes and to examine changes in body composition and performance. One case study of a swimmer with cerebral palsy (CP) concluded that while small changes in body fat levels did not impact performance, the muscle content of the body did impact performance. For those dancers with a limited range of movement in some parts of the body, muscle content may be different from able-bodied dancers, and lower in areas with reduced mobility. Each dancer is unique, and guidelines are not yet available for protein intake, but keeping to the guidelines from Chapter 5, together with adequate energy, represents the best option for now unless there is a medical need to limit protein intake.

There has also been some work looking at which formula for predicting basal metabolic rate will give the most accurate data for paralympic athletes in three groups: visual impairment, CP and limb deficiency. The Mifflin equation (see Chapter 3) was most accurate for those athletes with visual impairment, and the Owen equation for those with CP and limb deficiency (Juzwiak et al., 2016). Numbers are relatively small; there were 30 athletes total, but both males and females were included. Knowing that metabolic requirements, at least for this group, could be estimated by formulae devised in able-bodied individuals is a useful guide to nutritional requirements. Of course, the types and extent of disabilities are vast, and a spectrum not black and white, and consideration of whether there is an increased requirement or no change (or possible even a reduction) in requirements for specific nutrients and/or energy intake is needed on an individual basis. And disabilities are not necessarily static – some may not change over time, while others alter.

Body composition is a major driver of nutritional requirements – bodies with a higher muscle content have an increased requirement for energy and protein compared with bodies with a lower muscle content. Higher body fat levels have less impact on nutritional requirements as body fat is less metabolically active than muscle.

IV Altering body composition: when might it be helpful and how to approach making change

It would seem to be common sense that dancers aiming to be, or who are already, performing professionally simply need their body to be healthy and be able to carry out the movements they request of it, to a standard that an audience will enjoy. However, globally, there are still reports that this is not the case.

Pressure to be thin

Dancers from some disciplines, notably ballet, have over the last few decades faced pressure to have a particular 'look'. This 'look' for females has typically been medically on the border of underweight, bringing with it health risks. For males, the pressure may be more to look very lean but also strong. In other genres, the focus is generally on the quality of dance without criticism of body composition. Most, if not all, dancers are very aware of their bodies, and often highly self-critical. Some dancers are naturally lean: if they naturally have body fat levels at the lower end of the normal range and are meeting their nutritional needs, then their body will function healthily, and for them this is sustainable. Other dancers who are not naturally as lean as they feel they need to be, risk their health and wellbeing trying to be at a weight where their body fat levels are too low for their health. One reason frequently given for wanting female dancers to be thin is that male partners have to lift them. But male dancers are well aware that a taller, slim but strong dancer, who is aware how she can use her body in the lift, may in fact be considerably easier to lift than a smaller, lighter dancer who is not as skilled in what will reduce the work for her male partner.

There is more awareness that dieting is a risk factor for disordered eating, which many involved in dance including dance health organisations and organisers of competitions are aware of. Unfortunately, there are anecdotal reports that dancers are under pressure from teachers and coaches to supply incorrect information on health screening forms for competitions, which further risks their well-being.

Dancers who respond to the pressure to be thinner than is right for their body by restricting their energy intake will face all the risks of RED-S that are discussed in Chapter 11. If a dancer has gained body fat because their current diet is high in ultra-processed foods, includes little fruit and/ or vegetables and is low in protein, and that dancer adopts a more performance-appropriate diet there may well be changes in body composition. But if a dancer's diet is already focussed on lower fat proteins, wholegrain carbs, good portions of vegetables/salads, two to three servings of dairy or a good equivalent, plus necessary fats, with rare inclusions of high-sugar/high-fat snacks, then there is little or no room for manoeuvre in trying to reduce body fat without risking both physical and psychological harm. Activity can be reviewed as dance is not necessarily the best fitness training. Many dancers will undertake strength and conditioning as part of their training and preparation for performance and this can benefit their metabolism. But any type of exercise without adequate nutrition is not recommended.

Set-point theory and appetite regulation

There is much discussion over the concept that the body has a natural weight band that it will return to if food intake is adequate but not excessive. Research into the area is difficult in humans because in many countries there is a huge variety of food from minimally to highly processed, schedules that can make it hard to eat regularly and/or be active regularly, and at times, food is used for psychological rather than physiological reasons, all of which interfere with appetite regulation. In follow-up work on the study by Ancel Keys that started in 1945 on semi-starvation and re-feeding, most of the subjects overshot their original healthy weight after the study when they could eat normally again. Over time however almost all ended up back at their normal weight. There are no data available as to what any differences might have been between those who settled back at their previous normal weight and the small number who didn't. A review paper by Harris in 1990 concluded that: 'the level at which body weight and body fat content are maintained represents the equilibria achieved by regulation of many parameters'. This is echoed in other papers. Regulation of food intake is complex. There are mechanisms which signal the body to stop eating at the end of a meal, and mechanisms which regulate when hunger is felt again after the last meal or snack. Several areas of the brain are involved, and the drive to eat is impacted by metabolism, the nervous system and hormones including gut hormones like ghrelin, a short-term regulator, and leptin, which acts more over longer time frames (Hall et al., 2022). Trying to actively change body composition is a major challenge as the body is so well set up to keep itself stable.

Fact: Dieting is a risk factor for disordered eating

Fact: Appetite regulation is a very complex process which drives you to meet your nutritional needs

Fact: A diet with a high proportion of highly processed foods is more likely to disrupt appetite regulation than a diet based on less processed foods – though including some highly processed foods is not an issue

Fact: Lack of sleep can cause over-eating: sleep is vital for recovery as well as appetite regulation

Changes in body fat levels

Dancers who wish to reduce their body fat content are urged to consider very carefully the risks and benefits of limiting their energy intake. Reduced aerobic capacity, glycogen depletion, diminished strength and muscular endurance are all real risks, as are muscle mass loss, reduced hormone production, poor vitamin and mineral status and poor sleep quality.

If you are aware that your body fat levels have risen due to temporary, unusual, circumstances with regard to food choices and activity your best option is to firstly see how your body responds when you revert back to your normal levels of activity and your normal food choices – assuming these meet your nutritional requirements. It is likely that over time your body will settle back to its normal composition. You may be tempted to try and speed the process up, but allowing the decision-making part of the brain to interfere with the finely tuned mechanisms which regulate nutrition is best resisted. If you are aware your diet does not include the amounts of protein and fat, and the amounts and types of carbohydrates – including fibre – that are recommended in previous chapters then it's definitely worth working on this in the first instance and seeing how your body responds.

Make sure you are getting enough sleep, as lack of sleep can interfere with appetite regulation. Also, make sure you are taking enough water: although hunger and thirst should be regulated separately by the brain, because food can supply water, and drinks can supply nutrients, being intuitively in touch with what the body needs can be challenging. Anecdotally dancers are aware that sometimes they may have eaten but not drunk anything, when in fact their body likely needed both nutrients and water.

If your current food and activity are appropriate, then deciding to create an energy deficit by either reducing carbs/fats or increasing energy used by increasing activity may work in the short term and result in weight loss. In the long term, you may need to continue to restrict your energy intake to stay with the lower body weight, or risk embarking on a see-saw of body composition changes, and, potentially, disordered eating. Certainly, drastic reductions in food intake not only risk your energy and well-being but also bring a strong likelihood of unsustainability and the chances of ending up over-focussed on food and in a fight with your body over the drive to eat versus the drive to have less body fat. In addition, loss of weight is likely to include loss of muscle as well as loss of fat, which could impact on both metabolism and strength, although this can be mitigated by specific diet and exercise strategies.

If you are determined to try and reduce your body fat levels then seeking advice from a registered dietitian who has experience in working with dancers is advised.

Fad diets, which limit whole food groups, or drastically restrict intake on specific days, or for many hours of the day, are not appropriate for dancers. They increase the risks both of micronutrient inadequacies and low energy levels.

Increasing muscle content

Dancers who need to be stronger may see altered body composition, depending on the type of training they undertake. Strength training with an appropriate diet – increased protein with adequate energy – will result in increased strength, and may result in increased muscle volume.

How does food choice impact on body composition?

If your body doesn't get all the nutrients it needs it will signal this as hunger. Unfortunately, the signal doesn't necessarily guide you to specific foods for the nutrients you need. For example, lack of carbs is usually felt as a craving for sugar, which as a short-term solution may work but leaves you rapidly hungry again. Eating a range of grains, fruits, beans and lentils, some vegetables and some dairy/alternatives will provide both carbs and a range of other nutrients to contribute to your day-to-day requirements.

Food choices to help sustain healthy body composition

1   Eat regularly – you may have to adjust timings day to day, which is not ideal for appetite regulation, but your body gets what it needs.
2   Base your meals around the 1/3 plate principles unless you have an incredibly intense workload: around 1/3 plate of carbs, 1/3 protein, 1/3 plate veg/salad, with one to three tablespoons oils in cooking, in salad, from nuts or seeds or from avocado. Stir fries, grilling, baking, boiling, steaming and dry roasting (or with a small amount of oil) are the best options for day-to-day meals. For a very intense workload bring the veggies down to around ¼ plate and top up with more carbs. See the recipes section for more ideas.
3   Choose less processed rather than more processed options as a general principle: some processing is necessary and useful: bread and oatcake crackers provide a good range of nutrients, potatoes cannot be digested

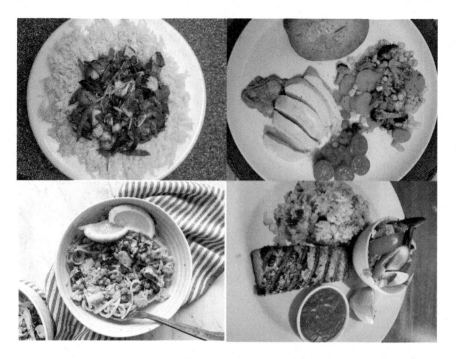

Photo 9.3 Balanced meals come in many formats, focus on variety from day to day.

when raw, cooking meat and fish reduces the risk of food poisoning and often improves palatability. Nut butters, with minimal additions, are useful to add some fats with protein.

4   Fruit and vegetables, meat and fish are great whether fresh or frozen. Canning reduces some nutrients but canned tomatoes, beans, lentils and fish are great options for the store cupboard. Some foods that have been dried, for example, pasta and rice are also very valuable nutritionally.

5   More processed products whether bought or homemade, such as cakes, biscuits and desserts, are hugely variable in the amount of nutrients they supply. Some can be a useful provider of a range of nutrients, whereas others are high fat high sugar with little protein or micronutrients. Comparing a slice of banana bread or other fruit bread especially if made with wholemeal flour, with a cupcake, or comparing Rich Tea biscuits versus cream-filled wafers reveal quite different nutrient profiles. Overall, these foods are not staples in the diet and are best kept to a small proportion of the meal plan. For training and performance remember that a 3:1 ratio of carb:fat (g) will supply the balance of nutrients your body needs. But it's good to keep in mind as well that highly processed foods are both enjoyable and often part of social situations, and this is an important part of any performer's meal plan.

6   Sugar is a carbohydrate, and as such can be used for energy in the body. But it lacks any other nutrient, which limits its value when there is a need to include so many other nutrients in the diet. Foods high in added sugar are likely to be lower in micronutrients, less filling and more likely to cause unwanted swings in blood sugar unless timing is carefully considered. In contrast, fruit is more useful as the natural sugars come with many micronutrients and phytonutrients, as well as fibre. Looking at foods that contain both fruit and added sugars can require a little more thought to decide how useful it will be for energy and appetite regulation. A product such as fruit yoghurt may have varying amounts of added sugar, but identifying how much from labelling is a challenge. Ingredients are listed in descending order, which can help, but the amount of sugar listed will be the total of the natural sugars from the fruit and the yoghurt, plus the added sugars. Best is taking plain yoghurt and adding your own fruit, or otherwise opting for those with higher rather than lower protein contents.

7   Highly processed foods that are served without vegetables or snacks that are often low in protein and/or high in fat are best kept to a minimum. This would include pot noodles, nuggets, sausage rolls (meat or vegetarian options), crisps, processed meat products and foods that rely on artificial flavours for taste.

Overall focussing on variety, including a good proportion of plant-based foods with adequate protein, and including less processed rather than more processed foods for the majority of your intake is a great way to allow your body to be at its best for training and performances.

V Resources

Nutrition (teamusa.org)
Intuitive eating by Evelyn Tribole and Elyse Resch, 4th Edition 2020.
'Just Eat It' Dr Laura Thomas/'How to Just Eat It' Dr Laura Thomas 2019/2021.

VI Learning outcomes

After reading this chapter the dancer should be able to:

1   Identify the elements of fitness relating to dance.
2   Describe the different compartments used in considering body composition.
3   Review techniques of measuring body composition and their limitations.
4   Explain factors that can impact on appetite regulation.

References

Berger, A.A. et al. (2011) Surprising evidence of pelvic growth (widening) after skeletal maturity, *Journal of Orthopaedic Research*, 29(11), pp.1719–1723.

Borga, M. et al. (2018) Advanced body composition assessment: From body mass index to body composition profiling, *Journal of Investigative Medicine*, 66(5), pp.1–9.

Hall, K.D. et al. (2022) The energy balance model of obesity: Beyond calories in, calories out, *The American Journal of Clinical Nutrition*, 115(5), pp.1243–1254.

Harris, R.B. (1990) Role of set-point theory in regulation of body weight, *The FASEB Journal*, 4(15), pp.3310–3318.

Huseynov, A. et al. (2016) Developmental evidence for obstetric adaptation of the human female pelvis, *Proceedings of the National Academy of Sciences*, 113(19), pp.5227–5232.

Juzwiak, C.R. et al. (2016) Comparison of measured and predictive values of basal metabolic rate in Brazilian paralympic track and field athletes, *International Journal of Sport Nutrition and Exercise Metabolism*, 26(4), pp.330–337.

Mitchell, S.B. et al. (2016) The role of puberty in the making and breaking of young ballet dancers: Perspectives of dance teachers, *Journal of Adolescence*, 47, pp.81–89.

Mitchell, S.B. et al. (2017) Understanding growth and maturation in the context of ballet: A biocultural approach, *Research in Dance Education*, 18(3), pp.291–300.

Sawyer, S.M. et al. (2018) The age of adolescence, *The Lancet Child & Adolescent Health*, 2(3), pp.223–228.

Terzis, G. et al. (2012) Muscle strength, body composition, and performance of an elite shot-putter, *International Journal of Sports Physiology & Performance*, 7(4), pp.394–396.

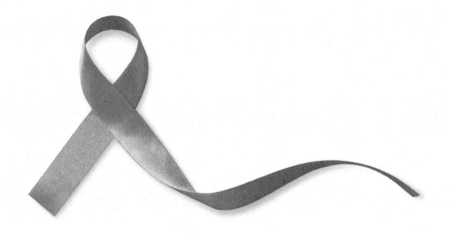

Photo 10.1 Early recognition, support and treatment give dancers the best change of a good recovery from disordered eating.
Photo credit: Chinnapong/Shutterstock.com

10   Disordered eating

Contents

Eating disorder myths and truths

Eating disorders myth	Eating disorders truth
Eating disorders are a choice	Eating disorders are serious and complicated mental illnesses, caused by a number of factors.
People never fully recover from an eating disorder	Eating disorders usually require specialist treatment, and it can take months or even years to recover fully, but it is possible for a good proportion of those who have had an eating disorder diagnosed to make a full recovery.
People with eating disorders are always underweight	Many people with an eating disorder are at a normal or higher weight. You can't tell if someone has an eating disorder just by looking at them
Men don't usually suffer from eating disorders	Although a higher proportion of sufferers are women, anyone can suffer from an eating disorder
Eating disorders are diets that have gone wrong	While a weight loss diet is well recognised as being a trigger for eating disorders, eating disorders are much more complex than a diet taken to extremes.

DOI: 10.4324/9781003219002-10

I Introduction

First and foremost, food is your fuel. Biologically you need to meet your needs. Food also plays an important part in most people's social lives; eating with others has many benefits, as well as being an opportunity to celebrate together often with specific foods for special occasions. While food will improve the emotions caused by lack of food – such as irritability and anxiety due to hunger – food cannot make a lasting change in feelings, if those feelings are due to what is happening in life rather than hunger. Everyone needs to eat, and different foods supply different nutrients. Society often divides foods into 'good' or 'bad', 'healthy' or 'unhealthy' but nutrition is not black and white, and a range of foods are needed to meet nutritional needs. Trying to live only or mainly on broccoli (usually seen as 'healthy') would result in malnutrition, as would trying to live only or mainly on chocolate (often seen as 'unhealthy'). Previous chapters cover the recommended proportions and amounts of nutrients that will set you up to dance at your best, when compared to not getting the right amounts, but remember also that your dance schedule is an important factor in your choice of foods. It is the types and amounts of food that make your diet more suitable – 'healthy', or less suitable – 'unhealthy', rather than trying to label individual foods. There are many different combinations you can put together that will meet your needs, and also work for your individual requirements and preferences – it is important for your well-being that you enjoy your food. Anxiety, stress and guilt about the food you eat suggest your relationship with food is challenging and worth addressing. If you have a medical condition that requires you to avoid certain foods or nutrients it will require more attention and means you have to focus more on food than other dancers. This area is covered in more detail in Chapter 13.

II Why do eating disorders matter?

Eating disorders are serious medical conditions. They affect mostly teenagers and young adults but can affect all ages, and those from all backgrounds. Sadly they have one of the highest mortality rates of any psychiatric disorder so need to be taken very seriously.

While people tend to think of anorexia nervosa (AN) and bulimia nervosa (BN) when eating disorders are mentioned, the reality is that atypical eating disorders are in fact the most common eating disorder diagnosis currently. The different categories of eating disorder are discussed in more detail shortly. There are treatments available for all eating disorders. If you are struggling with food/body image but think you are not ill enough to have treatment there is a useful book, 'Sick Enough' by Dr Jennifer Gaudiani, an eating disorders expert, that can be helpful.

Eating disorders result in risks to health both short term and long term. There is concern that fertility may be impacted in women. The risk of osteoporosis is increased: if periods stop bone density may be affected, and it is

recognised that this occurs from early on, and after six months of amenorrhoea (no periods) bone density is likely to be significantly reduced (Biller
et al., 1991). As bone density normally increases until the age of about 30
for many younger dancers low bone density can be improved with improved
nutrition and being at a healthy weight. When hormone levels are too low,
which in females may result in menstrual periods stopping, or becoming
more irregular, lighter and/or shorter (oligomenorrhoea) for months or
longer there is an increased risk of stress fractures. Males can also suffer
reduced hormone levels with a potential impact on bone health. Eating disorders bring an increased risk of gastrointestinal (digestive) problems and
finally, but extremely importantly, a dancer who is suffering from an eating
disorder is at risk of becoming detached and isolated, and are likely to find
that it affects the artistic side of performance as well as the physical side.

III Normal and appropriate eating versus disordered eating and eating disorders

The terms 'appropriate' and 'normal' are used in this chapter because the
eating patterns dancers can fall in to may be typical for their situation, but
may or may not be the most useful patterns from a nutritional perspective.
One aim of this chapter is to try and identify the factors that distinguish appropriate eating from disordered eating. For dancers there are many eating
patterns that can develop that are not going to result in effective, enjoyable
fuelling. Schedules may mean either very short breaks, or erratic breaks,
so it may be difficult to eat enough at lunch time. This is compounded if
the dance work after lunch is intense, as digestion will be slowed down,
and also it can be difficult to move freely when digesting a meal. Practice
does help – the gut can adapt, but careful planning is needed to get enough
nutrition in at the times available. This can mean snacks are used rather
than meals. While snacks are very useful, they often don't provide the balance and range of nutrients that a meal would. Timing of both meals and
snacks is a major challenge for dancers across their careers and in every
dance genre. The ability to change meal timings and still stay in touch
with appetite is a challenge, and well worth working to find your own best
solution to maintain energy and health. If money is an issue, then trying
to prioritise food can be difficult and can result in patterns of eating that
are not optimal, though not disordered either. Dancers can still experience
pressure to achieve a particular look or may feel there is an expectation to
do this, and this can lead to deciding that they need to restrict food below
requirements.

There are a few questions to think about when trying to work out what
normal and appropriate eating for a dancer looks like:

- *Is normal eating for a dancer having three balanced meals per day and one
  to three snacks?*

This is a great schedule, but if your schedule means that sometimes you have to have several larger well-planned snacks rather than a meal and snacks, that's OK too.

- *Is normal eating for a dancer eating when time allows?*

Yes, dancers often have very tricky schedules and may need to eat unconventional times – but this is not disordered eating. The important goal is that in 24 hours you put in what you need, without getting behind, as evenly spread as can be done within your schedule to avoiding being overly hungry or too full at any point in the day, and having good energy levels.

- *Is normal eating for a dancer eating when hungry and stopping when full?*

This is a great way to eat – but sometimes back-to-back classes or long rehearsals mean you have to eat earlier than you would like, in order to have the energy you need for the upcoming workload. So eating before you are hungry may be necessary – better this than getting to the level where your concentration and energy are compromised by hunger. It is also normal to eat more than you need at times – this will balance out if you are able to listen to your appetite on the days afterwards.

- *Is it normal/healthy for dancers to be tracking macros/calories?*

For those with no issues with food tracking macros and/or calories can be useful in the very short–term to help identify whether or not you are meeting your estimated requirements, although for energy (calories) needs your energy levels and hunger are generally a good guide if you respond to the signals your body sends. Checking your protein intake, or the balance between fats and carbs may be useful, but it's not necessary or advisable to do this for more than a few days just to get a range of data to be able to then adjust your intake if needed. It can be the start of the slippery slope into disordered eating: if you find yourself focussing overly much on the numbers then best not to track at all – focus on food rather than numbers.

- *Is normal eating for a dancer to be neither restricting nor binging?*

This is the aim: being able to meet your body's nutritional needs with a variety of enjoyable foods. Remember that while your mind can help you to make balanced choices, your body is responsible for signalling to the brain when you have eaten enough. When you are very hungry you might crave high sugar foods, to get a quick energy hit, but in many circumstances your body may benefit more by having a balanced meal or snack, maybe with some high sugar food if that feels right.

What is an eating disorders – some definitions

One widely used definition of an eating disorder is that it is: 'a persistent disturbance of eating or eating-related behavior that results in the altered consumption or absorption of food and that significantly impairs physical health or psychosocial functioning' (DSM V, 2013).

It is important to also note that the disturbance in eating is not caused by a medical or another psychological problem. For example, if people have a digestive problem they may eat less to feel less pain, or if they are depressed they may have no appetite, and no motivation to eat, but this isn't an eating disorder. Sometimes of course people, including dancers, may have more than one illness simultaneously. It's important if you do struggle with food and have another medical or psychological problem that those who you get support from are aware of your full history to be able to help you effectively.

The UK eating disorders association, Beat, has stated that eating disorders are:

> Serious mental illnesses that involve disordered eating behaviour. This might mean restricting food intake, eating very large quantities of food at once, countering food eaten through purging, fasting or excessive exercise, or a combination of these behaviours. It is important, though, to remember that eating disorders are not about food. Instead, the eating behaviour might be a coping mechanism or a way for the sufferer to feel in control.

Eating disorders are difficult to treat, and recovery is hard work and often takes many months or more. The sooner treatment starts the better the outlook for recovery, so if you are struggling with and eating disorder, or disordered eating its best to get help as soon as possible. If you are a dance student, then your college or university may have resources available to help you; explore what is available and ask for onward recommendations if needed. If you are a professional dancer, then it is best to explore all the options you can access from the healthcare you have available: identifying a specialist who is adequately trained to treat dancers may take a little longer but is likely to be beneficial in the long run.

When to worry – screening tools and warning signs

The SCOFF questionnaire was devised by eating disorder specialists in 1999 (Morgan, Reid & Lacey, 1999) to be a quick screening tool, which can be used by doctors but also works for individuals. It was found to be valid and is a useful tool.

*The SCOFF questions**

Do you make yourself Sick because you feel uncomfortably full?
Do you worry you have lost Control over how much you eat?
Have you recently lost more than One stone in a three-month period?
Do you believe yourself to be Fat when others say you are too thin?
Would you say that Food dominates your life?
*One point for every 'yes'; a score of ≥2 indicates a likely case of AN or BN.

If you are worried that you may have an eating disorder, take the test and if it indicates you likely have an eating disorder it gives a starting point for discussions with your GP/primary care doctor. Even if you only score one point, unless it is in answer to weight loss, and there was a very good reason for the weight loss, and you answer 'no' to all the other questions this score is an indication that your relationship with food is troubling, and you would benefit from support. This is a quick screening tool, and there are other questions that are useful for you to ask yourself, such as whether you are regularly feeling guilty, anxious and stressed around food, and this is impacting on your food intake, or whether you are only allowing yourself to eat a small range of foods in order to feel in control. If the answer to either or both is yes then getting some support would be useful.

Let's now look at what others may see. Although the signs in Table 10.1 may indicate an eating disorder, any approaches need to be planned and thought through as there may be many other causes. If you have concerns then asking the dancer how they are is far better than assuming they have an ED. If there are several signs which make you fairly sure a dancer has an eating disorder, then it's still best to open a conversation that you are concerned for their well-being, and take the conversation from there. Having an eating disorder is not something anyone wants or chooses, but seeing a way out of it can often be very difficult. If you have a friend or colleague you have concerns about and you raise this with them, you may find they do not want to talk about it and/or deny it. It's best to be prepared for this. You cannot force anyone to get help, but you can reiterate your concerns for their well-being, and be supportive. Sufferers do appreciate this, even though it may not seem this way – if no one is saying anything, then they can

Table 10.1 Signs a dancer may have an eating disorder

Warning signs that a dancer may be suffering from an eating disorder for teachers, family and friends *Remember there may be other reasons for these signs, so enquiries need to be tactful*
Weight loss/weight fluctuations Poor/variable concentration Variable energy levels – more tired than others Variable mood Not eating as much as normal/expected Eating alone Choosing only limited low-calorie foods Avoiding social food, e.g. cake, snacks or meals with others More dizzy than normal/fainting Feeling cold all the time Wearing baggy clothes more than expected Exercising more than previously/needed

feel as though they must be fine, and how they are feeling/behaving is not a problem. It can take time for people to be ready to make changes, and sadly sometimes this doesn't happen voluntarily: compulsory treatment may happen for those at very low weight, as making changes when very starved is immensely difficult.

Types of eating disorder

Anorexia Nervosa: This is probably the eating disorder most associated with dancers, but the reality is more complicated, and most dancers with serious eating disorders will not have AN, nor necessarily be at low weight. Typical AN is an illness characterised by low weight, because AN usually involves severely restricting food intake. Atypical AN also exists, affects more people that typical AN, and sufferers will not be at very low weight. Excessive exercise and binge/purge cycles may be factors in someone's AN too. Some other possible signs of AN include:

* Distorted perception of weight – seeing the body as much bigger than it really is.
* Preoccupation with and/or fear of gaining weight.
* Obsessive behaviour such as counting calories.

Often people believe that they can't have AN if they are eating regular meals and snacks, but if these meals and snacks don't meet their needs, and weight loss is ongoing, with fear of healthy weight and preoccupation with food and weight this is still AN.

AN has many physical consequences which will eventually impact on the ability to dance, although initially performance isn't always affected. The physical consequences include:

* Lanugo hair – the layer of fine hair that can develop all over the body, but is often most noticeable on the back in AN.
* Hair loss: losing hair much faster than normal happens in malnutrition including in AN. It does reverse once nutrition improves.
* Hypothermia: low body temperature. Most people with AN struggle to feel warm unless rooms are very well heated.
* Hypotension (low blood pressure), bradycardia (low heart rate), poor circulation, fainting.
* Amenorrhoea: periods stop (in adult females not on 'The Pill').
* Osteopaenia or osteoporosis: bone density becomes abnormally low, or very low.
* Muscle weakness – eventually.
* Hyperactivity/fatigue: energy is limited, so although sufferers may feel very driven to do more than is asked of them, once activity can stop energy levels are extremely low.

- Irritability, rigidity, poor concentration and sleep disturbance: consequences of inadequate food.
- Anxiety, depression, aggression and isolation: also caused in part by inadequate food.
- Elevated blood cholesterol: this returns to normal when weight and nutrition improve.
- Increased gut transit time, constipation and abdominal pain: poor digestion can make it harder to try and increase food intake.
- Increased severity of viral and bacterial infections (Brown et al., 2008): although sometimes sufferers seem to get less symptoms than other people and possibly suffer fewer mild infections (Pomeroy et al., 1992), the low level of white cells often seen means the body struggles to fight off viruses and bacteria, so infections can be more difficult to recover from than expected.

It can be really useful to know that many of the symptoms listed above are mostly due to the effects of starvation. Starvation doesn't mean eating nothing – it happens when there is a significant gap between intake and requirements – for example, only getting 50% or so of the energy needed. In the study by the physiologist Ancel Keys in the 1940s where he restricted the food intake of healthy normal men to about 50% of their requirements there were profound physical, psychological and social changes. These changes, symptoms of starvation, include:

- Being preoccupied with food
- Tiredness
- Weakness
- Gastrointestinal discomfort
- Headaches
- Reduced tolerance to cold
- Impaired concentration, alertness, comprehension and judgment
- Depression
- Anxiety
- Irritability/apathy
- Reduced sense of humour
- Isolation

As well as this some of his study participants who mostly were only able to eat what they were given, also found that they experienced binges on occasions when they did have access to additional food.

Bulimia Nervosa: involves cycles of bingeing and purging, the frequency can vary. This means the sufferer will eat unusually large amounts of food in one go, beyond fullness and then engage in behaviour to compensate for the food eaten, such as making themselves sick, fasting, taking laxatives or excessively exercising. There will be significant emotional distress. It is important to note that taking laxatives results in dehydration and doesn't have any impact on energy intake. It can result in an empty feeling, but this will usually be accompanied by digestive problems and low energy levels.

BN has many physical consequences which will impact on the ability to dance. These include:

- Swollen salivary glands
- Periods may become irregular or stop in females
- Dental/gum problems if vomiting is occurring regularly
- Gastrointestinal problems, e.g., constipation
- Damage to the digestive system. This can result in reflux and damage to the oesophagus from vomiting, or damage to the large bowel from laxative over-use
- Electrolyte levels in the blood may become abnormal, which can impact on muscle function
- Hypotension: low blood pressure
- Oedema – fluid retention may be a problem
- Weight and mood fluctuations caused by big swings in fluid levels and nutrient availability
- Irritability, poor concentration, anxiety, depression, fatigue and sleep disturbances
- In severe cases there can be cardiac problems
- Muscle cramps

Binge eating disorder: involves bingeing, i.e., eating large amounts of food at once, but not engaging in compensatory behaviour associated with bingeing in bulimia or anorexia. Over time this often results in weight gain. Attempts to lose weight by restricting food intake then tend to precipitate further binge episodes.

OSFED: If someone's symptoms don't fit all the criteria for another diagnosis, they might be diagnosed with 'other specified feeding or eating disorder' (OSFED). Less commonly nowadays, you might hear the term 'eating disorder not otherwise specified' (EDNOS). An OSFED or EDNOS diagnosis does not mean that the eating disorder is less serious. This could be, for example, rapid weight loss with very restrictive intake though not yet underweight or, e.g., chronic dieters who monitor and control weight to prevent any increase. Also, those who compensate for only small amount of food or those who chew and spit large amounts of food.

Avoidant/restrictive food intake disorder (ARFID): ARFID is defined as an 'eating or feeding disturbance (including but not limited to apparent lack of interest in eating or food, avoidance based on the sensory characteristics of food, or concern about aversive consequences of eating), as manifested by persistent failure to meet appropriate nutritional and/or energy needs'. In this case, there are no worries about weight or shape that are impacting on food choices but could be, for example, a struggle with particular textures of food, or perhaps a fear of choking, or being ill after eating a specific food or group of foods that means that food intake is restricted with the consequences of signs and symptoms of malnutrition.

IV Incidence and prevalence of eating disorders amongst dancers

Eating disorders most commonly affect young people, particularly those in their teens and early twenties. They can and do however affect almost all ages from the very young to the very old. Eating disorders are more prevalent in those who are female, although males are estimated to make up around 25% of those suffering from an eating disorder.

The estimated prevalence of ED overall in the UK is around 2% (Beat, 2022). A meta-analysis by Arcelus and colleagues in 2014 concluded that the overall prevalence of eating disorders in dancers was 12%. The overall eating disorder prevalence rate for ballet dancers was 16.4%. Breaking this down he found that the prevalence of AN was 2%, higher in ballet dancers at 4%. The prevalence of BN was 4.4% overall and 2% in ballet dancers, and for EDNOS (now OSFED), the prevalence was 9.5% overall and 14.9% in ballet dancers.

What is also important to note is that dancers scored higher on the screening tests that had been used in the research, so were also experiencing more symptoms of disordered eating. This means that although they didn't have a full-blown eating disorder, nonetheless, they had less good relationships with food than non-dancers.

Overall dancers seem to have a higher risk of AN and OSFED than the general population, but don't seem to be at higher risk of BN. The overall risk is at least twice as high as for the general population.

As OSFED is the most common eating disorder diagnosis it can sometimes be difficult for dancers and those working with them to feel that the situation is serious enough to prioritise treatment as it isn't the well know AN or BN. But the distress experienced and the physical and psychological effects will impact on the dancers' training and performance, so treatment is necessary in the same way a dancer would seek advice and treatment on managing a physical injury, even if was not immobilising.

V Risk factors and protective factors

For many years it has been known that not everyone is at the same risk of developing an eating disorder. There are proven risk factors for eating disorders which can be divided into three main categories. These are biological risk factors which relate to genetic background, medical conditions or nutritional intake. Psychological risk factors again may be genetic or

Table 10.2 Risk factors for eating disorders in all athletes including dancers

Risk factors for eating disorders

Biological risk factors	Psychological risk factors	Social risk factors	Sport-specific risk factors
Having a close relative with an eating disorder	High achieving, Perfectionism	Weight critical environment	Dieting/low-weight environment/ an environment that emphasises thinness
Having a close relative with a mental health condition	Body image dissatisfaction	Experiencing bullying or abuse	Weight-related sport and aesthetic sports – judged partly by appearance
History of dieting	History of an anxiety disorder	Loneliness and isolation	Coach pressure
Negative energy balance – whether intentional or not	Low self-esteem	Family food issues (also psychological risk factor)	Injury/illness including depression
Type 1 Diabetes	Extreme competitiveness	Family discord	Abuse: previous/current
Early growth spurt	Highly self-critical	Trauma	Performance anxiety
	Reduced sense of identity as a person rather than as a dancer		Negative self-appraisal of athletic achievement

related to life experiences. Social risk factors relate to your experiences with other people whether your peers or those who are in a teaching or management role. Table 10.2 summarises eating disorder risk factors for dancers.

Dancers have the additional issues of weight/shape, for example, pas de deux/double work involving lifts. Working in studios with mirrors can be a challenge for some dancers who may struggle to use the mirrors constructively to guide technique, and may instead become overly focussed on body shape.

It is now thought that people have a predisposition towards an eating disorder, which would be one or more risk factors shown in Table 10.2, and then, they experience a trigger, which precipitates the eating disorder. The trigger could be trauma, bereavement or a stressful life event such as moving away from home, difficulties in a significant relationship, being under pressure for important exams. While the trigger may be something life-changing this isn't always the case. It might be something that would seem small to another person, but this doesn't mean that the outcome is small – eating disorders are always significant. No one chooses to have an eating disorder, and sometimes there is no obvious cause. Rather than looking to blame someone or something it's better to focus on how to access help to start the, often challenging, road to recovery.

When it comes to getting treatment, historically there have been challenges to dancers receiving consistent support to access psychological treatment. Dancers often struggle to 'fit in' treatment and may find that insufficient priority is given. Treatment for an eating disorder or other mental health problem needs to be given as much priority as a physical 'injury'. Finally, professional dance is a career where there is both a lack of control over many areas of the work and also for many a level of job insecurity, which is not helpful for those at risk of eating disorders and disordered eating, because EDs often serve as a coping mechanism.

Protective factors

Research by those working in the field of eating disorders in sport has identified a number of factors that protect athletes – and likely dancers – from developing eating disorders (e.g., Bratland-Sanda & Sundgot-Borgen, 2013). These are:

1   A positive, person-oriented coaching style rather than a negative, performance-oriented coaching style.
2   Social influence and support from team-mates with healthy attitudes towards size and shape.
3   Where there are coaches who emphasise factors that contribute to personal success such as motivation and enthusiasm rather than body weight or shape.
4   Where there are coaches and parents who educate, talk about and support the changing female body.

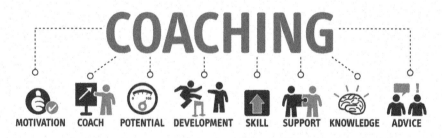

Photo 10.2 Positive coaching styles help protect against against eating disorders.
Credit Trueffelpix/Shutterstock.com

5   The presence of an atmosphere where early treatment is supported: athletes rarely self-identify with eating disorders, so those working with the athlete, such as their coach, need to be more pro-active than with other medical problems.

VI Managing food and treatment options for eating disorders

Although eating disorders result in a change in eating habits and food intake, making changes to food is only a part of what needs to be changed for recovery to occur. In fact, if the change is only to food, then the dancer is likely to experience other problems, as the use of food has been in response to something psychological, rather than nutritional. It might seem that fixing food should fix the eating disorder, but it is essential to do the necessary psychological work as well, to understand the role the eating disorder is playing and find ways to cope in a way that isn't harmful to well-being in any way. This psychological support may be with a suitably qualified and experienced therapist or psychologist and is likely to take the form of sessions weekly for a number of weeks. There are a number of different approaches, and ongoing research helps to identify those which are most useful. Sometimes group treatments are offered rather than individual therapy, and sometimes both may be used. Family therapy can be useful, depending on circumstances.

Restricting versus intuitive eating

As you saw earlier, normal eating for anyone, including a dancer, is not an easy thing to define. What is easier to identify is whether someone is restricting or experiencing binges. When there is a thought process that limits the amounts and/or types of food that is eaten to less than the body needs, this is restricting. To be able to eat intuitively is the aim, with adjustments for schedules which mean that eating can't just be exactly when we would like. Intuitive eating is only possible if eating has been adequate. If food has been restricted appetite will not be reliable, as the body is driven to try and restore nutrients. Appetite may be erratic, and the experience of hunger/ satiety (fullness) may be confusing. For this reason, meal plans are typically used in the treatment of disordered eating and eating disorders.

Meal plans

Meal plans based on three regular meals and one to three snacks are widely used in the treatment of eating disorders. Meals will normally include appropriate amounts of all food groups: good sources of protein, carbohydrate-rich foods, fruit/vegetables/salad, plus some oils or good sources of fat. To get the best range of nutrients, food needs to be varied, and changes made progressively to increase variety, remembering that no one food is intrinsically 'good' or 'bad'. It is the amounts and frequency of different types of foods that determines whether an overall diet is 'healthy' or not. Variety is important across all food groups, as is the ability to be flexible with food choices. Different types of bread, grains, protein sources and fat sources are all important. Being able to include butter, oils, spreads and nut/seed butters without anxiety is an important part of recovery but may need support from a specialist dietitian to work out a suitable time frame for changes, to avoid either trying to go too fast and ending up overwhelmed, or the whole process taking many months, with long gaps between challenges, which is likely to make the process more difficult overall.

Recovery for those below their biologically appropriate weight requires weight restoration. Dance adds to the challenges of this situation, as there are still pressures on some dancers to look a particular way, which usually involves being thinner than normal and below their normal healthy weight. This is a very difficult and contentious area and if you are experiencing this, then getting support from an appropriate impartial person or organisation is strongly recommended. For the brain and body to recover fully, it is important to restore muscle and fat to healthy levels. Trying to stay below where the body needs to be is likely to mean not recovering fully from the eating disorder. This area is likely to require careful guidance from those with experience in treating eating disorders. Experience of experts in the field has shown that, in recovery from low weight, an average rate of weight gain of around 0.5 kg per week works optimally (Royal College of Psychiatrists, 2005). Although some people are able to recover at a faster rate of weight gain, for many it can be hard work to achieve steady weight restoration, as it requires consistently giving the body nutrition above and beyond what feels comfortable to provide the nutrients to repair the body. Generally limitations on activity are needed; this will depend on the severity of the ED. Severe weight loss impacts not just on the obvious area of loss of fat and arm/leg muscle but can also affect the heart muscle. It is not unusual for those struggling to eat normally to also struggle not to over-exercise. If this isn't tackled then although food intake may improve, health may not benefit. Exercise patterns should be evaluated in those with ED to ensure is exercise is not being used in a problematic way. There can also be health consequences from exercise after purging, and again, exercise may need to be limited. These limits should always be tailored to the individual, and regularly reviewed.

Some dancers with eating disorders not at low weight are able to recover without the support of an intense daypatient or inpatient programme at a clinic, hospital, or other specialist treatment centre. Those at low weight may need more support.

Types of programme for eating disorder treatment

In the UK, there are three main options for the location and intensity of eating disorder treatment, although there is some overlap. The three are outpatient, daypatient and inpatient programmes, though may go by slightly different names, for example, referring to the level of intensity. In the US and other countries, they will potentially be slightly different, but there will still be more and less intense programmes.

Outpatients typically have regular (e.g., weekly) psychotherapy together with some dietetic input, which is overseen by a psychiatrist – a medical doctor who specialises in mental health. Outpatients have treatment that only takes place for a small number of hours each week. This treatment involves the least alteration to study or work plans.

Daypatients attend a hospital or clinic for several hours on a number of days per week. Typically at least one main meal and one snack is supervised at the treatment centre, and there are normally groups running through the day. Some daycare is from before breakfast until after the evening meal. This treatment does mean that changes have to be made to study or employment schedules.

Inpatient treatment is residential treatment, and is usually for a minimum of two weeks, although more typically stays are 6–12 weeks. All meals and snacks are supervised and there will be a variety of therapy groups and 1:1 sessions during the days. As with any hospital stay, this requires time out from work or studies. After inpatient treatment, there will often be a period of stepdown daycare before moving back to outpatient care.

Which treatment option is advised depends on several factors. Unfortunately, the availability of treatment varies according to location: some areas of the UK, for example, have very little provision for eating disorders and there are very limited beds in general. This can mean that even when more intense treatment, daycare or inpatient, would be the most useful option, sufferers are managed as outpatients until more support is available. In the UK, those who have private medical insurance may be able to access treatment more quickly than waiting for NHS treatment, but insurance companies typically only cover a limited amount of dietetic support and therapy. As it is often easier to make quicker progress to recovery early after an eating disorder begins, we would urge anyone struggling to look for help as speedily as possible.

How to get help for eating disorders and disordered eating

If you are a dance student struggling with food a good starting point would be to speak to either your GP/primary care physician, or to support staff at your school/college, if there is a student services department. They may advise you to speak to your GP, or they may be able to provide access to some support directly. If you are feeling physically unwell as a result of your behaviour around food, then medical help is advised. Either see your GP, or, if you are feeling acutely unwell due to very poor food intake or vomiting/ using a lot of laxatives, then you are advised to access emergency services by phone/in person.

Professional dancers based in one location are advised to contact their GP for advice, or emergency services if necessary. If you are touring and need help, your best option will depend on your situation, although tele-health may well be an option. If you feel extremely unwell, then we advise you seek urgent help. If you are medically and psychologically stable, then it may be ok to wait to see your GP. 'Beat' in the UK, or national eating disorder associations in other countries have details of how to best access support. If you have private medical insurance, it is worth seeing what this might cover, but it usually requires a GP referral in any case. Check how much treatment is covered as if it's only a very limited number of sessions you might then need to transfer to an NHS team.

VII Resources

www.beateatingdisorders.org.uk.
Book: 'Sick Enough' by Dr Jennifer Gaudiani.
Book: 'Heal Your Relationship with Food' by Juliet Rosewall et al. (2020).
Book: Overcoming Binge Eating: Chris Fairburn (2014).

VIII Learning outcomes

After reading this chapter the reader should be able to:

1 Explain the consequences of eating disorders for dancers.
2 Discuss factors that can prevent dancers from developing eating disorders.
3 Summarise appropriate eating behaviours for dancers.

References

Arcelus, J., Witcomb, G.L. and Mitchell, A. (2014) Prevalence of eating disorders amongst dancers: A systemic review and meta-analysis, *European Eating Disorders Review*, 22(2), pp.92–101.
https://www.beateatingdisorders.org.uk/get-information-and-support/about-eating-disorders/how-many-people-eating-disorder-uk/?gclid=CjwKCAjw3K2 XBhAzEiwAmmgrAhX3NzT3KpGxYl7LWw87UznD9bW3KWEyi_L6UArDi Cnm1AnhSUyrqRoCnKsQAvD_BwE
Biller, B.M. et al. (1991) Osteopenia in women with hypothalamic amenorrhea: A prospective study, *Obstetrics and Gynecology*, 78(6), pp.996–1001.

Bratland-Sanda, S. and Sundgot-Borgen, J. (2013) Eating disorders in athletes: Overview of prevalence, risk factors and recommendations for prevention and treatment, *European Journal of Sport Science*, 13(5), pp.499–508.

Brown, R.F., Bartrop, R. and Birmingham, C.L. (2008) Immunological disturbance and infectious disease in anorexia nervosa: A review, *Acta Neuropsychiatrica*, 20(3), pp.117–128.

DSM V (2013) The diagnostic and statistical manual of mental disorders, *American Psychiatric Association*, 5th Edition.

Morgan, J.F., Reid, F. and Lacey, J.H. (1999) The SCOFF questionnaire: Assessment of a new screening tool for eating disorders, *BMJ*, 319(7223), pp.1467–1468.

Pomeroy, C., Mitchell, J.E. and Eckert, E.D. (1992) Risk of infection and immune function in anorexia nervosa, *International Journal of Eating Disorders*, 12(1), pp.47–55.

Royal College of Psychiatrists (2005) Guidelines for the nutritional management of anorexia nervosa. Council Report CR130, July 2005.

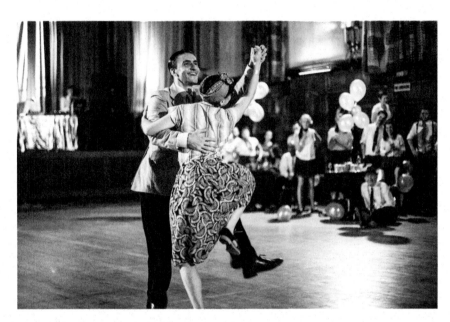

Photo 11.1 Nutrition can play a role in injury risk reduction to allow dancers to perform at their best.

Credit: Photo courtesy of Helen Rimmell

11 Health and performance

Contents

I Anxiety, creativity and dance performance

Every dancer is unique, and this includes their genetics, family background and life experiences. Both in training and as an occupation, dance can bring a significant amount of uncertainty, and unpredictability. Both during training and if employed in a company dancers may not be guaranteed roles in performances, and the roles they are allocated can change at very short notice. For some dancers, this may be very exciting, and it can open up unexpected opportunities; for others, this may bring stress and result in anxiety. Some will navigate the many challenges dancers face without psychological stress, while others may struggle. There is a lack of data on the number of dancers who have accessed psychological support from a psychologist, psychotherapist or counsellor, whether a dance specialist or not, but it is likely that many dancers will have benefitted from appropriate and timely psychological support. Accessing suitable support can be a challenge, although moves to online treatment have opened up options, particularly for those moving between different locations.

From a mental health, perspective nutrition has a role in mood and psychological well-being as well as in energy levels. This is not to suggest that food can fix all psychological problems, but there is certainly value in exploring the impact of different nutrients on mental health. And while a diet

DOI: 10.4324/9781003219002-11

that meets the body's needs can't prevent mental health problems, a diet that doesn't meet needs can lower mood and energy.

Research by May et al. (2020) demonstrated that creativity can be enhanced by appropriate training. The brain requires energy to function, and significant under-fuelling, where energy intake doesn't meet requirements, will result in impairments to concentration, comprehension, alertness and judgement, as well as mood being lower (Tucker, 2006). Undertaking more research into the effects of poor nutrition on creativity is challenging as it is not ethical to ask participants to compromise their energy intake and health over the longer term, so research is typically undertaken either over a short period of time, or participants are studied over time to find links between their nutrition intake and areas of health and well-being. There are some specific nutrients that can impact on mood which it is useful to consider.

Research has found that in the short-term carbohydrate is helpful for challenging cognitive tasks (Mantantzis et al., 2019). Cognitive tasks involve acquiring knowledge and understanding through integrating thoughts, experiences and information received via the senses. Learning dance choreography would be an example. Identifying longer-term effects of choice and adequacy of carbs is less easy, but Knuppel et al., identified adverse effects of sugar intake from sweet food/beverage on long-term psychological health (2017).

Anecdotally many people find that if they eat just high-sugar food over a period of a few hours their body reacts with good energy for a short period of time, but energy may then dip, and hunger kicks in again. As sweet snacks typically lack protein and micronutrients, there is then a risk of not getting enough of the nutrients the body needs to perform effectively. Also, swings in energy can mean you struggle to be at your best when dancing. Highly processed foods, including high-sugar foods, are likely to lack the B vitamins needed for the nervous system to function properly and are less good for the gut microbiome. As the gut microbiome can impact positively on the brain, there may be benefits if dancers can include foods which support the gut. There is already some research evidence of potential benefits, although more work is needed (Margolis et al., 2021).

Although relying on high-sugar foods may mean you find sustaining creative dance practice is less easy than it could be, this does not mean that using sweet foods to boost energy at strategic points in performances is a bad plan. At times it may be your best strategy – and Chapter 4 explores this in more detail. Making sure you take in all the other nutrients you need is essential however to get the most out of this strategy.

Knowing that energy, mood and concentration are all impacted by nutrition your best approach is to aim to meet your needs for both macro- and micronutrients with three meals and at least one snack per day, meals should include a good portion of protein, enough carbs, oils or spreads in cooking, on bread or on salad, and some veggies or salad. Including two or three portions of fruit daily will give additional benefits – see Section III below. Snacks can be just fruit, or fruit can be part of some or all snacks, depending on energy needs.

Foods that can support mood

Nutrients/types of food/drink to include regularly to support mood	Examples of foods
Foods/drinks that support good gut bacteria	Live yoghurt, Fermented foods, e.g., sauerkraut, kimchi, kefir, kombucha
Omega 3 fats	Oily fish, algal oil, rapeseed oil, walnuts, flax seed
Iron rich food	Red meat, poultry, fish, beans and lentils, fortified cereals
Selenium	Brazil nuts, meat, fish, wholegrains
B group vitamins	Wholegrains, meat, fish, eggs, milk, yoghurt

II The female athlete triad and RED-S

To be a healthy dancer requires your system to have an adequate supply of energy. This sounds very obvious, and at one level it isn't complicated. But appetite regulation can be challenging in a busy schedule, when hunger and breaks may not coincide, and increasing workloads can make it difficult to meet requirements. Add in an increased risk of disordered eating due in part to aesthetic demands in Western dance culture, plus financial and resource constraints and there are a number of scenarios where dancers can fail to take in enough energy.

The female athlete triad (the triad) refers to the links between levels of energy availability, menstrual function and bone mineral density (BMD). The concept has been around for a number of years, with research to back up the concepts (De Souza et al., 2014).

Figure 11.1 shows the three components of the triad and the spectrum that each component covers.

Low-energy availability (LEA) may or may not be linked to disordered eating or an eating disorder. Functional hypothalamic amenorrhoea (FHA) is the situation where females have no periods (or only artificial periods due to the oral contraceptive pill [OCP], which are not the same as having natural periods). Bone health is impacted by hormone levels: low hormone levels can result in low-bone density. Each of the three aspects of health is a spectrum, for example, a dancer may have levels of low-energy availability, menstrual periods may be irregular rather than missing altogether, and bone density can be low, in a range known as osteopaenia, which is below the normal range but not yet as low as osteoporosis. There are clear clinical cut-off points identifying where the osteopaenic range transitions into osteoporosis (Table 11.1).

While for females not on the OCP it is relatively easy to track whether periods are regular, irregular or non-existent, unfortunately, there is no easy

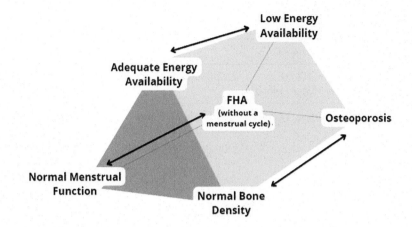

Figure 11.1 The three components of the triad, and the spectrum that each component covers

Table 11.1 The areas of health in the female athlete triad

Female athlete triad	Partial triad	Healthy female dancer
Low-energy availability	Reduced energy availability	Adequate energy availability
Amenorrhoea	Irregular periods/low hormone levels	Normal periods/hormone levels
Osteoporosis	Low-bone density	Normal bone density

way to identify what is happening with bone density other than having a
DEXA scan. DEXA stands for dual-energy X-ray absorptiometry, and a
DEXA scan uses a very low dose of X-rays to measure bone density, which
is painless and takes only a few minutes. The results will show whether areas
measured, usually the hip and lumbar spine, are in the normal range, or in
the osteopaenic or osteoporotic ranges. Low-bone density increases the risk
of bone fractures as bones are more fragile than they should be.

Once menstrual periods have stopped for several months, or weight is sufficiently low and energy availability has been low, bone density will be affected.
The good news is that bone density is not fixed, and restoring hormone levels
will help improve bone density at least to the age of around 30. Bone density
normally increases until about the age of 30 years before it plateaus for a few
years and then starts to decrease. For men, this decrease is steady and gradual
throughout their lives. For women, there is a faster drop after the menopause,
around the age of 50, before the rate of bone loss settles to a level similar to that
of men. Unfortunately, while weight-bearing exercise and physical activity are

normally very useful for increasing bone density, this is only the case if hormone levels are normal and energy availability is adequate. The same applies to nutrients which are important for bone health. The nutrients most dancers will associate with bone health are calcium and vitamin D. Alongside these there are a number of additional nutrients which are important for normal bone formation. These include protein, vitamin K, vitamin C, phosphorous, magnesium, copper, zinc and selenium. Weight-bearing exercise and an adequate supply of nutrients combined with adequate energy availability will give dancers strong bones. How strong does depend on genetic factors too, as osteoporosis is known to run in families (Pouresmaeili et al., 2018).

Dancers have been shown to be at risk of the triad, with a small study finding 40% of elite female ballet dancers experiencing low-bone density, irregular periods and reduced energy availability (Doyle-Lucas et al., 2010). Improving nutrition and ensuring workload is not excessive can improve energy availability and allow regular periods, which in turn will allow bone density to improve, depending on age.

Relative energy deficiency in sport (RED-S) is a more recent concept, and so is less well researched. RED-S includes the areas addressed by the Triad but looks at other body systems and applies this to both males and females. The authors of the RED-S consensus statements from 2014 and 2018 (Mountjoy et al., 2014; Mountjoy et al., 2018) define the basic principle of energy availability for athletes, which from a physiological point of view include dancers, as:

$$\text{Energy availability (EA)} = [\text{energy intake (EI) (kcal)} - \text{exercise energy expenditure (EEE)}]/\text{fat-free mass (FFM) (kg).}$$

Using fat-free mass means that most dancers won't easily be able to see if they do have adequate energy availability, as there is no way to know your current fat-free mass without having it measured. For ways to accurately measure body composition, see Chapter 9.

RED-S can occur for a number of reasons. It can be that a dancer had adequate energy available until their workload went up. Then, possibly due to lack of time, and/or a schedule that crossed mealtimes and made judging food needs difficult, or possibly due to disordered eating, that dancer wasn't able to increase their energy intake to cope with the increased workload and moved into energy deficiency. It could also be that workload hasn't changed, but other circumstances change, such as finances or physical or mental health problems impacting on appetite, resulting in reduced energy intake. While the reasons a dancer finds themselves in energy deficiency are important and will need addressing to allow energy intake to increase, the potential consequences of RED-S are the same.

The consequences of RED-S can affect the whole body. The systems affected are shown in Table 11.2, with the potential impact on training and performance shown in Table 11.3.

A detailed review of how relative energy deficiency impacts on body systems is covered in the International Olympic Committee (IOC) consensus statement on relative energy deficiency in sport (RED-S): 2018 update (Mountjoy et al., 2018).

Table 11.2 Body systems affected by RED-S

Menstrual function
Bone health
Endocrine
Metabolic
Haematological
Growth and development
Psychological
Cardiovascular
Gastro-intestinal
Immunological

Table 11.3 Potential impact of RED-S on training and performance

Increased injury risk
Delayed recovery from injury
Decreased training response
Decreased endurance performance
Decreased muscle strength
Decreased glycogen stores
Depression
Irritability
Decreased concentration
Decreased co-ordination
Impaired judgement
Increased risk of illness
Increased digestive issues

Source: After Mountjoy et al. (2018).

One area not addressed in detail in the Triad or RED-S is that of body fat levels. Body fat is essential for health and normal physiological function. Body fat is usually designated either 'essential' or 'storage', but the term 'essential' isn't very helpful here, because it is also essential to have some storage fat. Women have around 12% essential fat, while men have around 3% essential fat. This fat is found around organs of the body, such as the kidneys and heart to protect against damage. In addition, the minimum amount of storage fat is a little more for women than men. As discussed in Chapter 9, healthy levels of body fat for young males are from 13% to 20%, though some male dancers can be healthy with lower natural body fat levels, even some below 10%. For young women, healthy levels of body fat are regarded as around 17–25%. Some female dancers may naturally have slightly lower levels and still be healthy, but this will not be typical. Body fat levels do normally rise slightly with age.

RED-S is a relatively new area of research. It currently suffers from a lack of standardisation as to how LEA and the negative health outcomes are assessed (Logue et al., 2018). This should improve over coming years. There is already a screening tool for females, the Low Energy Availability in Females (LEAF) questionnaire, which has been shown to be useful in assessing whether young female athletes are experiencing the effects of low-energy availability (Luszczki et al., 2021). More data on adult athletes and dancers are needed. There is also a new questionnaire and interview protocol for males which may be useful for male dancers but again more data is needed (Keay et al., 2018). A further questionnaire, the DEAQ (Dance-specific Energy Availability Questionnaire), has been trialled on-line and may be useful (Keay et al., 2020) once clinical validation has been completed.

Dancers who suspect they are suffering the impact of low-energy availability are advised to seek support to improve health and performance, including medical assessment and individualised nutrition advice from an experienced registered dietitian.

Checklist for Dancers: RED-S risk self-management

Risk of RED-S	Reduce the risk	Suggestions
Appetite reduced after exercise	You can train your gut as you can your dance muscles, and work towards always meeting your requirements.	Start with small snack straight after dance. Have a meal as soon as possible after that.
Workload suddenly increased	Carry extra snacks and items to top up meals you bring with you to dance.	Varied bars, nuts and dried fruit, oatcakes all travel well.
Previous food issues	If you start to struggle meeting your requirements seek professional help quickly.	Dance specialist therapists or psychologists can provide support: OneDance UK and IADMS have directories.
Challenges to food resources e.g. time/budget	Planning meals/snacks makes best use of time & money. Check financial support available.	Cook several portions of meals and freeze if possible. Bulk buy in a group to save money. See Chapter 12.

III Injury risk reduction, recovery from injury and staying well: a nutritional perspective

While the risk of injuries related to dance can be reduced by, and for, dancers, it is very difficult to prevent injuries completely. To avoid dance injuries altogether probably means not dancing, so the next best option seems to be to assess how the risks of injury can be reduced. When it comes to data on dancers and their injuries, a large-scale, very thorough survey, 'Fit to Dance 2', was carried out by One Dance UK in 2002, as a follow-up to their initial survey in 1993 (Laws 2005). 1,056 dancers responded to the 2002 survey. While some of the perceived causes of injuries may have been addressed over the last two decades, taking a look at these causes and the links with nutrition is a good place to start when thinking about how nutrition can contribute to injury risk reduction.

In Fit to Dance 2 (FtD2), types of injuries were divided into five categories: muscle, joint, bone, tendon and other. The 'other' category covered a wide range of injuries including psychological injury. The location where injuries occurred was explored – whether in class, rehearsal, performance or outside dance, and the anatomical location was also recorded. Perhaps most importantly the perceived cause of injuries was reported. Fatigue and over-work were perceived to be the cause of 38% and 37% of injuries respectively. Because dancers were asked to rate each potential contributing cause to injury as either often, sometimes or never there may be an overlap between

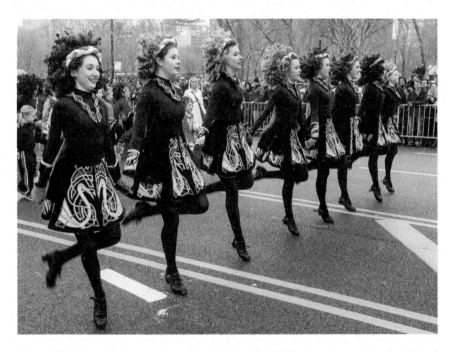

Figure 11.2 Nutrition strategies to reduce the risk of fatigue can reduce the risk of injury, which is recognised as high in Irish dancers.
Source: Credit Kobby Dagan/Shutterstock.com

these two causes. While overwork is not directly linked to nutrition, there is certainly a link between fatigue and nutrition. Though the best nutrition cannot prevent the dancer becoming fatigued, certainly inadequate nutrition can result in early fatigue. If the schedule doesn't include enough time to eat or drink or the dancer experiences LEA, then that will add to the risks of injury. Of note, 6% of dancers reported the perceived cause of their injury to be inadequate diet.

In a more recent survey of over 1,000 Chinese dancers carried out online, the same questions were asked of Chinese dancers who danced predominantly Chinese folk dance and Chinese classical dance, with smaller proportions whose dance style was ballet or contemporary dance. This survey also found fatigue and overwork were given as two of the four main perceived causes of injury. From a nutritional perspective over 50% reported using weight-reducing eating plans and over 25% reported having psychological issues with food, 21% reporting an eating disorder (Dang et al., 2020).

Thinking about avoiding injuries, a great starting point is to use nutrition strategies to minimise the risk of fatigue. Strategies to minimise the risk of fatigue include:

1   Maintaining good hydration. Taking fluid regularly, even in a very busy schedule, is worth it, particularly when energy levels start to drop. For times when breaks are possibly shorter than usual a water bottle of suitable size (typically at least a litre), that you refill regularly will make keeping on top of hydration more practical – Chapter 7 gives more detail.

2   Planning for the workload: although schedules can, and do, change, make sure that you have access to enough food for meals and snacks. If eating normal size meals isn't easily possible due to schedules, then eating smaller amounts frequently will optimise energy levels. Thinking about the level of intensity of your schedule, the timing and length of breaks will help your choices on types of carb – slower or faster acting, the need to divide food across the breaks that you have. If you have a lot of high-intensity work soon after eating you may feel more comfortable opting for lower fibre choices, though some dancers have no problems with this.

3   Including foods naturally rich in anti-oxidants. These anti-oxidants may reduce the cell damage caused by reactive oxygen species which are produced in response to exercise in the body. Polyphenols, plant-based compounds particularly found in berries, apples, grapes and pears, act as powerful natural anti-oxidants. Unlike supplements of anti-oxidant vitamins which can hinder repair processes in the body, polyphenols are helpful and they can be considered valid nutritional support against oxidative stress caused by physical activity (D'Angelo & Rosa, 2020).

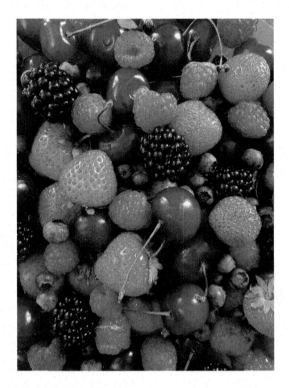

Figure 11.3 Fruits rich in polyphenols.
Credit: I.Irinka.Photo/Shutterstock.com

More information about polyphenols is covered in Chapter 12. Although green and black tea and red wine are often highlighted as containing polyphenols, the caffeine in the tea, and alcohol in wine do not make these the best options for increasing polyphenol intake. Extra virgin olive oil is one of the few sources of fats that will supply useful amounts of polyphenols but is only useful if it is affordable, and then only for use in suitable meals. Focussing on including two to three portions of a variety of fruits daily for polyphenols will bring other nutritional benefits and seems the best strategy for most dancers (Figure 11.3).

After an injury – are there specific nutrients that can help with recovery in the early stages?

When any part of your body is injured a sequence of events is set into motion. Your body initiates an inflammatory response which can last up to several days. Swelling and soreness are often experienced and are normal. Along with this, you produce oxidants including free radicals, which can damage cells and are a normal part of the injury recovery process.

Anti-oxidants in your body will combat free radicals, but recovery may be more efficient if you ensure you include foods with anti-oxidant and anti-inflammatory properties, for example, fruits//vegetables and oils rich in vitamins A, C and E (see Appendix A for more information), and in plant polyphenols, for example, some fruits, particularly cherries and berries, this area is looked in more detail in Chapter 12. One research example is that dancers who supplemented their diet with tart cherry juice did see evidence of more speedy recovery from exercise that damaged muscle fibres (Brown et al., 2019).

Omega-3 fatty acids are involved in combating inflammation – see Chapter 6 for more information on these.

Inflammation is a process that is not all negative; the inflammatory process plays an important role in wound healing and positive adaptation to exercise. Dancers need to balance the need to reduce inflammation in the short term to be able to train and perform, with the negative impact on healing and adaptation from using foods and supplements which reduce inflammation (Owens et al., 2019).

Nutrient focus after injury to specific body tissues

When looking at the information on nutrition for specific types of injury there is another factor to keep in mind. If you need to use crutches or have an injury that limits day-to-day mobility as well as your ability to dance, then it is likely that your normal daily activities will use more energy than usual, and/or you may be limited in the food you can prepare. If surgery is planned and you have the space, then preparing meals in advance and freezing them are good options. It's fine to mix in some ready meals if these work for you, though if you can add some veggies or a small side salad that will increase your intake of antioxidants. Meal deliveries can range from those with a good portion of protein, carbs and veggies with some fats, to a high-fat, highly processed meal with little or no veg. Focus on the former and minimise the latter if you do need to include a number of these for a while when recovering from injury – or if you are using them for any other reason, such as a really busy period in your training or work schedule.

It is important to note that after an injury, there is inflammation and the body is under stress. You can need between 15 and up to 50% or more additional energy to recover from injury, depending on the extent and severity; the highest increases are after burns (Smith-Ryan et al., 2020). This needs to be compared against how much more you would use if you were normally active. While a small reduction in total energy intake may be appropriate to avoid significant changes in body composition when activity is reduced due to injury, this should be managed and monitored carefully where possible; dancers after significant surgery or injury may not need to adjust their energy intake at all. Aiming for a protein intake of at least 2 g/kg body weight after injuries seems the best strategy currently (Frankenfield, 2006).

Spreading this protein out over the day, including 20–40 g per meal depending on your total intake for the day, with the remainder in snacks will mean you can be in positive protein balance, with a steady supply of protein for your body to use for recovery. As you saw in Chapter 5, foods rich in the amino acid leucine are useful for repair, because leucine is a great stimulator of muscle protein synthesis, and many injuries will include muscle damage.

Dental or oral surgery can limit the textures of food you can eat, and occasionally only liquids or purees are possible. If this is expected to continue for more than 24 hours then it is worth exploring the range of medical supplement drinks – such as the Ensure, Fortisip, Aymes, Nualtra and Complan ranges. It is much harder to meet your requirements with liquids/pureed food than with regular meals and snacks.

Muscle injuries and nutrition

Muscle is mainly made of protein. Muscle strains are where muscle fibres are over-stretched or torn. Recovery time will depend on the severity of the injury but can be up to several weeks, or even months. During this time it makes sense to pay particular attention to protein intake and how it is distributed over the day. There is a lack of data that increasing protein intake can reduce the severity of muscle damage in injuries. But there is some evidence that increasing your protein intake after an injury can minimise muscle loss due to not being able to maintain normal muscle use and may optimise the repair process. Close et al. (2019) have suggested it may be helpful for injured athletes to aim for 2.3 g protein/kg body mass per day and to divide this fairly evenly over the day. This is a very high protein intake and will be a challenge to many dancers. If 2.3 g/kg body weight is more than double your normal intake then aim initially for at least 1.6 g/kg body weight consistently and then try and increase to at least 2 g/kg body weight. Vegetarians may find this a challenge, but it is just as important for those on plant-based diets. Main meals should each have at least 20 g protein, and closer to 40 g in one serving may be useful after a muscle injury. Previously research suggested that there was little value for muscle synthesis in having more than 20 g protein in one meal or snack for maximum muscle benefit. More recently, Macnaughton et al. (2016) showed that 40 g could be used when resistance exercise involved the whole body. See Chapter 5 for more information on this.

When you are thinking about your intake of carbs and fats after a muscle injury, any changes to normal requirements will depend very much on how the injury impacts on dance activity. Healing uses energy; the amount is going to vary, with more severe injuries using more energy in repair. Most dancers will aim to continue exercising the parts of the body not impacted by the injury. Being under-fuelled will impact on recovery from injury, so taking note of hunger and responding with nutrient-dense food is the most useful way of optimising recovery.

There is a link between muscle injury recovery and vitamin D, so check you are following guidelines for vitamin D. Although you can make vitamin D during summer months if you get adequate sunlight exposure, many dancers use higher factor sunscreen or sun block, or may cover up, which, while preventing the skin from being damaged, may reduce or prevent vitamin D synthesis (Passeron et al., 2019). Aim for just 10–15 minutes of sunlight exposure for arms and legs between 11 a.m. and 3 p.m. with lower factor sunscreen for the time of exposure, on most days of the week. Use suitable sunscreen for all other times in the sun. If adequate sunlight exposure isn't possible then continuing with vitamin D supplements all year round is likely to help you avoid vitamin D deficiency.

Polyphenols, a type of phytonutrient, have been suggested to help with recovery from muscle damage. Along with including a good range of fruits and vegetable in your diet, some specific options may be useful in helping recovery from muscle damage. For example, Tart cherry juice has been shown to accelerate recovery from exercise-induced muscle damage (EIMD) in females (Brown et al., 2019). Berries of all types are another good source of polyphenols.

One final option to consider is the use of creatine monohydrate after injury. Creatine is examined in more detail in the supplements chapter (Chapter 8), as it is often used by those looking to improve strength and lean mass. With regard to injury, one small study where creatine was given in a simulated rehabilitation process for a leg that had been in plaster, showed that muscle area and power increased more quickly with creatine versus placebo (Hespel et al., 2001). A further study using creatine while one arm was in plaster, showed that loss of arm muscle was less with creatine compared with placebo. Again numbers were very small, and the study was carried out in healthy young men, normal activity not stated (Johnston et al., 2009). Nevertheless, if your diet is already good and you face some time with a limb completely immobilised, creatine is worth considering. Close et al. (2019) suggest 20 g/day for five days followed by 5 g/day after that.

Joint injuries and nutrition

Dancers are prone to joint injuries and some dance styles are more prone to specific joint injuries, for example, ankle injuries for Irish dancers. As most dancers are aware, joints are complex structures where two or more bones meet and are held together by ligaments to give the body structure. To allow movement in joints other structures are needed, including ligaments, cartilage and synovial fluid. Tendons connect bones to muscles so can be found attached via muscle to bones.

Joint injuries that affect dancers include dislocations, fractures, sprains and strains, overuse injuries such as tendonitis, arthritis and low-bone density (osteopaenia and osteoporosis). The nutritional aspect of recovery from a joint injury depends on the type of injury. If it's a bony injury we will look at that next. If ligaments, cartilage or tendons are damaged, then ensuring you are meeting your protein and energy needs will give you the best chance of your injury healing as efficiently as possible. Your state of hydration is also worth considering, as dehydration reduces blood flow to tissues within the body (Trangmar & Gonzalez-Alonso, 2017) and may delay healing. Check fluid advice in Chapter 7.

Bone injuries and nutrition

As we saw in section II of this chapter, although most people are aware that calcium and vitamin D are important for bone health, many are not aware of the other nutrients necessary for healthy bones. Of the macronutrients, protein is directly needed for bone, but enough energy from carbs and fats is vital to fuel the process of normal bone turnover. For the micronutrients, phosphorous and magnesium are found in significant amounts in bone. Other minerals and vitamins needed for processes involved in bone health include potassium, fluoride, manganese, copper, boron, iron and zinc, possibly silicon, vitamins A, C, K and B group (Palacios, 2006). With this extensive list, if you have a bone injury, whether it's a stress fracture, a fracture or following surgery to bone, a nutrition review to check you are including foods rich in all of these is a useful strategy. When dancers are injured it can feel like they have less control of life than usual. Nutrition is one area where the dancer can contribute to their recovery by making sure their nutrition is as good as it can be – though remembering there is no one perfect diet. Use Appendix A to check out the foods containing micronutrients that are helpful for bone health. Many dancers will be able to include foods that are good sources of these. Those who either need to follow a restricted range of foods for medical or other reasons or have limited access to foods due to their budget or living situation may need to take a once-daily multivitamin/mineral with 100% of a wide range of micronutrients until they are able to access a wider range of foods.

Nutrition and tendons, ligaments and cartilage

Vitamin C is essential for collagen synthesis which is found in cartilage, tendons and ligaments. Because your body can't store surplus vitamin C, there is no point in taking it in large doses, but making sure you include a range of fruits and vegetables, including some from berries, citrus fruits, peppers and tomatoes, peas and cabbage will make sure you have an adequate supply of vitamin C.

Copper deficiency will also cause the reduced synthesis of collagen. Shellfish, liver, cocoa, nuts and seeds and quinoa are good sources of copper. If you are able to include some of these foods regularly, then copper deficiency is unlikely, and additional copper is not beneficial.

Small studies in athletes suggest that gelatin may be helpful to decrease injury rates and reduce recovery time from injuries by increasing collagen synthesis (Shaw at al., 2017, McAlindon et al., 2011).

Other injuries and nutrition

Bruising is not uncommon in dancers and results in damage to red blood cells. Useful nutrients to pay particular attention to if you have experienced significant bruising are protein, iron, zinc, vitamin B12, folic acid, vitamin C and vitamin K, as well as making sure energy needs are met. In addition, seek medical advice on how best to manage the bruising with cold and/or heat and/or compression and rest if necessary.

Although psychological injuries do come into this category, the area of disordered eating and eating disorders is covered in detail in Chapter 10. A range of other psychological issues were reported in the FtD2 report, including anxiety, low self-confidence, tiredness and burnout, depression and stress. Nutrition and mood are discussed in Section 1 of this chapter. From a nutritional perspective those suffering with anxiety are best to limit their intake of caffeine, as high intakes can contribute to anxiety (Smith, 2002). Regular adequate balanced meals will minimise the risks of anxiety from low blood sugar levels and hunger. There can also be nutritional causes for tiredness. These include low intakes of iron, vitamin B12 and/or folate, lack of fluid, and under fuelling – whether it be from inadequate carbs, or possibly fat, or a low protein intake making muscle repair and development less likely. Burnout and stress are more likely to result in nutritional deficiencies than cause them, as self-care is unlikely to be prioritised in times of high stress.

Returning to dance after injuries, holidays and other absences: managing DOMS

Returning to dance after a break, whether this is for holiday, injury or another reason gives an opportunity to review and if necessary reset food and fluid strategies. Does your fluid intake need more focus? Are you meeting protein and carb targets? How are you doing with fruits and vegetables? How is your calcium intake? Iron-rich foods? A quick check on these and a commitment to gradual change if necessary can enable you to feel more secure that you are supporting your body returning to dance. Of course, the first days back after a break can be a challenge as well as the joy of returning to the activity that gives you joy. Delayed onset muscle soreness – generally known as DOMS – is frequently part of those first few days back. Most, if not all, dancers are familiar with DOMS, which you typically feel from around 24–48 hours after unusually strenuous activity, which could include returning to dance after a holiday or break following injury depending on the workload undertaken. Currently, there is a lack of evidence around the link between adequate fuelling and experience of DOMS, but Molaeikhaletabadi et al. (2022) showed that low-fat chocolate milk after 90-minute training sessions reduced DOMS as well as improving recovery in a small group of university badminton players. It is good practice to take in adequate amounts of both protein (e.g. 20–40 g) and carbs after training to refuel effectively and this may have a role in minimising DOMS.

A review by Kim and Lee (2014) concludes that caffeine does reduce DOMS, though the dose of 5 mg/kg body weight 1 hour before and 24 hours after exercise (Hurley et al., 2013) is the equivalent of around three cups of coffee in one go and will be above the single dose maximum advised by the European Food Safety Authority (EFSA, 2015). You will need to assess whether this is a wise or practical option, also depending on your tolerance to caffeine.

Omega-3 fatty acids have also been trialled for reducing DOMS. Different doses have been trialled, which makes comparison difficult, but Kim and Lee (year) suggest that taking 1.8–3 g of omega-3 fatty acid may be effective in reducing DOMS after exercise.

Taurine and branch-chain amino acids (BCAA) have been shown to reduce DOMS, but studies are small, not in elite athletes or dancers, and background protein intakes aren't defined. So while you may wish to consider taking additional taurine and/or BCAA, it isn't yet clear if there would be any benefit, and your priority is better to be consistently achieving your protein goals.

Tart cherry juice, berries, beetroot and pomegranate have been shown to have some impact on DOMS in dancers. A review by Bongiovanni et al. (2020) also found that creatine monohydrate and vitamin D appear to provide a prophylactic effect in reducing EIMD rather than DOMS specifically. They comment that β-hydroxy β-methylbutyrate, and the ingestion of protein, BCAA and milk could represent promising strategies to manage EIMD, but that dancers are advised to only make stepwise changes to their diet rather than combining two or more options. And of course you would want to make sure your day-to-day diet is as good as it can be before spending on products that may be expensive.

Staying well

Dancers and athletes who are highly active can find that their immune system works less effectively and they have more frequent infections. There is evidence from athletes that higher levels of infections are seen when training intensity increases. Meeting nutrient requirements minimises this risk, but exceeding requirements hasn't been shown to help (Williams et al., 2019).

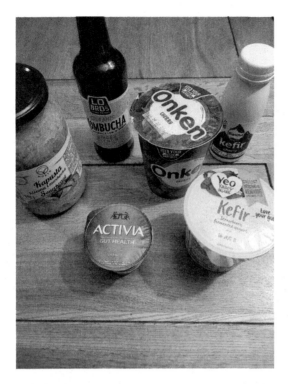

Photo 11.2 Probiotic foods.

Check Table 11.4 for nutrients which are needed for your immune system to work optimally. As well as the nutrients listed, enough energy from carbs and fats is also essential. Staying hydrated is useful for many reasons, one of which is it maintains saliva flow and enzyme content which are part of your immune system (Fortes et al., 2012).

Lack of rest and sleep can also reduce how well your immune system works. High stress levels will also negatively impact on your immune system – this is recognised in sport though more research is needed in dance.

Prebiotics and probiotics that support your gut bacteria may be useful for your immune system and well-being. Foods containing natural probiotics include fermented foods such as live yoghurt, sauerkraut, kimchi and fermented berries.

Beware claims for any food or supplement that can 'boost' your immune system: your aim is to have a normally functioning immune system – this is not a situation where more is better.

Avoiding getting sick is only partially under your control. Good hand hygiene and making sure you follow food safety guidelines will minimise the risk of a number of infections that can be transmitted via surfaces or food.

Table 11.4 Nutrients and foods for the immune system

Nutrient	Good food sources	Role
Protein	Meat/chicken/fish/eggs/ cheese/tofu/pulses/Quorn	Essential for white cells
Vit A	Orange/green veg and fruit, dairy, egg yolk	Protects epithelium and mucus integrity; enhances immune function
B group vitamins	Many protein foods, wholegrains, some dairy products	Immune cell regulation
Vit C	Many fruits and vegetables	Supports functions of both acquired and innate systems
Vit D	Fortified foods, oily fish, egg yolk Supplements usually needed	Stimulates innate immunity, enhances antimicrobial response
Selenium	Brazil nuts, seafood, eggs, lentils	Supports innate and acquired systems
Zinc	Meat, seafood, green vegetables and seeds	Supports innate and acquired systems, e.g., epithelial function, microbe death
Iron	Red meat, liver, chicken, dark chicken meat, oily fish seafood, eggs, grains, pulses, nuts and seeds, fruit and vegetables	Involved in functions of both innate and acquired systems: inflammation can also impact iron levels
Magnesium	Green leafy vegetables, nuts, bread, fish, meat and dairy products	Connection with both innate and acquired immune systems
Fibre	Wholegrains, fruit and veg, pulses	Can modulate the microbiome

IV Pregnancy

Pregnancy is a time where nutrient needs change – and this starts even before conceiving. Dancers considering pregnancy are advised to make sure they have a good intake of folic acid. Some countries fortify some flour, for example, non-wholemeal flour, or other foods, with folic acid. General advice is to take a supplement of 400 µg of folic acid daily up until 12 weeks of pregnancy; check the current advice for the country you are living in. Even if folic acid isn't taken before conception it's still advised to take up until 12 weeks of pregnancy. A good intake of folic acid in the early stages of pregnancy can reduce the risks of neural tube defects such as spina bifida. In addition, try and include foods rich in folate (the natural form of folic acid)

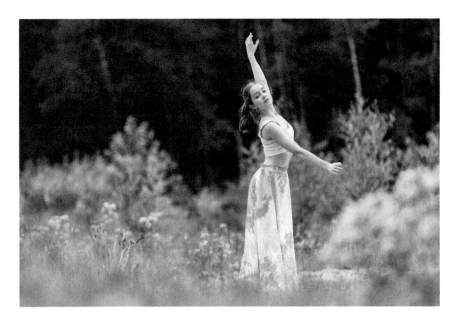

Photo 11.3 Vitamin D levels can be improved by time outside in summer months (follow safe sunlight exposure guidelines).
Source: Photo courtesy of Robert Biesemans

such as green leafy vegetables, beans, peanuts, sunflower seeds, wholegrains and also breakfast cereals with folic acid added to them. There are a small group of people who may be advised to take a higher dose of folic acid; this includes those with diabetes or are on anti-epilepsy medication. Any dancer with a long-standing medical condition considering pregnancy is advised to check with their GP whether they need the higher dose.

Make sure any supplements you take are suitable to be taken in pregnancy. This includes vitamin and mineral preparations, for example vitamin A is not advised in pregnancy.

There are a number of foods which are not advised in pregnancy. As this can change slightly from time to time please use this list as a guide and check for any recent changes with your GP or a reliable source. Caffeine advice has changed over time; currently, the maximum recommended by most countries is 200 mg per day which is about two cups of coffee or two to three cups of tea. The table of caffeine content of food and drink in Chapter 8 gives more detail. Herbal tea is best kept to a maximum of four cups per day.

Foods to avoid include: Unpasteurised milk and anything made from it such as unpasteurised goats cheese, but ordinary cheese from pasteurised milk is fine to include in your diet.

Cheese with a mould rind such as Brie or Camembert.

Any kind of pate or game meat. Cold sausage-type meat such as chorizo and salami are safest if cooked.

Any undercooked meat or poultry. Undercooked duck, quail or goose eggs.

Raw or undercooked eggs unless you are certain they don't bring a risk of salmonella.

Raw fish, raw shellfish and uncooked smoked fish. Swordfish, marlin, shark, Limit oily fish to twice per week and limit tuna to twice per week.

Unwashed fruit, vegetables or salad.

Liquorice root.

Alcohol.

Morning sickness

Morning sickness is nausea, and sometimes vomiting, that affects some women significantly and others not at all. It can also impact at any time of day, and not necessarily in the morning although that is typical. Morning sickness is common in the early weeks of pregnancy, but usually resolves by week 16–20 of pregnancy. A small minority of women continue to experience morning sickness for the duration of pregnancy.

There are strategies that can help with morning sickness. The nutritional suggestions are:

- Eat something like dry toast, crispbread, low-fat cracker(s) or plain biscuit(s) before you get out of bed.
- Eat small, frequent meals, similar to the normal dance nutrition advice: good proportion of carb, protein, veg/salad and lower fat rather than higher – avoiding fried foods, pastries and rich sauces. Plain food is often tolerated best. Include regular snacks, so you eat something every two to three hours.
- Eating cold foods rather than hot ones may help as cold food smells less.
- Sipping fluids little and often, rather than in larger amounts in one go, may help prevent vomiting. Trial different drinks to see which are most palatable. It may help to keep food and fluids separate – drinking up to 30 minutes before a meal and then from an hour after a meal.
- Eat foods or drinks containing ginger – there's some evidence ginger may help reduce nausea and vomiting – but check with a pharmacist before taking ginger supplements during pregnancy.
- Getting enough rest is also helpful, as tiredness can worsen nausea.

Changing requirements

There is a lack of data on energy and nutrient requirements for pregnant dancers and athletes. What is clear is that energy needs will increase gradually over pregnancy; although, rather than 'eating for two', the increased requirement by the end of the third trimester is likely to be the equivalent of the addition of a substantial snack, such as a sandwich, or a bowl of yoghurt, granola and fruit per day. Requirements will vary on the amount of dance that is undertaken as pregnancy progresses. Modifications to the dance workload that can be undertaken are likely to be needed due to the changes in body shape and centre of gravity. In the first few weeks of pregnancy energy needs will be very similar to a dancers normal requirements, providing these have been adequate with no level of restricting. Making sure meals and snacks are evenly spread out will help maintain blood glucose levels and also energy levels. Any dancer starting pregnancy at low weight will likely be advised to make sure that weight gain is adequate, and potentially more than for women who start pregnancy at a normal weight.

Fluid continues to be important, with slightly increased fluid needs in pregnancy, though pressure on the bladder as the baby grows can make this more of a challenge. Aim to maintain a good urine output and avoid dehydration and overheating.

V Resources

Mountjoy, M. et al. (2018) International Olympic Committee (IOC) consensus statement on relative energy deficiency in sport (RED-S): 2018 update, *International Journal of Sport Nutrition and Exercise Metabolism*, 28(4), pp.316–331.

De Souza, M.J. et al. (2014) 2014 Female Athlete Triad coalition consensus statement on treatment and return to play of the female athlete triad: 1st International conference held in San Francisco, California, May 2012 and 2nd International Conference held in Indianapolis, Indiana, May 2013, *British Journal of Sports Medicine*, 48(4), p. 289.

Returning to Sport/Dance restoring Energy Availability in RED-S? – BJSM blog – social media's leading SEM voice (bmj.com).

VI Learning outcomes

After reading this chapter the reader should be able to:

1   Discuss the links between food and mood.
2   Review the relationship between the female athlete triad and RED-S.
3   Explain the potential consequence of RED-S on a dancer's performance.
4   Summarise nutritional strategies a dancer could consider after injury.

References

Bongiovanni, T. et al. (2020) Nutritional interventions for reducing the signs and symptoms of exercise-induced muscle damage and accelerate recovery in athletes: Current knowledge, practical application and future perspectives, *European Journal of Applied Physiology*, 120(9), pp.1965–1996.

Brown, M.A., Stevenson, E.J. and Howatson, G. (2019) Montmorency tart cherry (*Prunus cerasus L.*) supplementation accelerates recovery from exercise-induced muscle damage in females, *European Journal of Sport Science*, 19(1), pp.95–102.

Close, G.L. et al. (2019) Nutrition for the prevention and treatment of injuries in track and field athletes, *International Journal of Sport Nutrition and Exercise Metabolism*, 29(2), pp.189–197.

D'Angelo, S. and Rosa, R. (2020) Oxidative stress and sport performance, *Sport Science*, 13, pp.18–22.

Dang, Y., Koutedakis, Y. and Wyon, M. (2020) Fit to dance survey: Elements of lifestyle and injury incidence in Chinese dancers, *Medical Problems of Performing Artists*, 35(1), pp.10–18.

De Souza, M.J. et al. (2014) 2014 female athlete triad coalition consensus statement on treatment and return to play of the female athlete triad: 1st International Conference held in San Francisco, California, May 2012 and 2nd International Conference held in Indianapolis, Indiana, May 2013, *British Journal of Sports Medicine*, 48(4), p.289.

Doyle-Lucas, A.F., Akers, J.D. and Davy, B.M. (2010) Energetic efficiency, menstrual irregularity, and bone mineral density in elite professional female ballet dancers, *Journal of Dance Medicine & Science*, 14(4), pp.146–154.

Fortes, M.B. et al. (2012) Dehydration decreases saliva antimicrobial proteins important for mucosal immunity, *Applied Physiology, Nutrition, and Metabolism*, 37(5), pp.850–859.

Frankenfield, D. (2006) Energy expenditure and protein requirements after traumatic injury, *Nutrition in Clinical Practice*, 21(5), pp.430–437.

Hespel, P. et al. (2001) Oral creatine supplementation facilitates the rehabilitation of disuse atrophy and alters the expression of muscle myogenic factors in humans, *The Journal of Physiology*, 536(2), pp.625–633.

Hurley, C.F., Hatfield, D.L. and Riebe, D.A. (2013) The effect of caffeine ingestion on delayed onset muscle soreness, *The Journal of Strength & Conditioning Research*, 27(11), pp.3101–3109.

Johnston, A.P. et al. (2009) Effect of creatine supplementation during cast-induced immobilization on the preservation of muscle mass, strength, and endurance, *The Journal of Strength & Conditioning Research*, 23(1), pp.116–120.

Keay, N., Francis, G. and Hind, K. (2018) Low energy availability assessed by a sport-specific questionnaire and clinical interview indicative of bone health, endocrine profile and cycling performance in competitive male cyclists, *BMJ Open Sport & Exercise Medicine*, 4(1), p.e000424.

Keay, N., Overseas, A. and Francis, G. (2020) Indicators and correlates of low energy availability in male and female dancers, *BMJ Open Sport & Exercise Medicine*, 6(1), p.e000906.

Kim, J. and Lee, J. (2014) A review of nutritional intervention on delayed onset muscle soreness. Part I, *Journal of Exercise Rehabilitation*, 10(6), p.349.

Knüppel, A. et al. (2017) Sugar intake from sweet food and beverages, common mental disorder and depression: Prospective findings from the Whitehall II study, *Scientific Reports*, 7(1), pp.1–10.

Laws, H. (2005) *Fit to dance 2-report of the second national inquiry into dancers' health and injury in the UK*. Newgate Press, London.

Logue, D. et al. (2018) Low energy availability in athletes: A review of prevalence, dietary patterns, physiological health, and sports performance, *Sports Medicine*, 48(1), pp.73–96.

Łuszczki, E. et al. (2021) The LEAF questionnaire is a good screening tool for the identification of the female athlete triad/relative energy deficiency in sport among young football players, *PeerJ*, 9, p.e12118.

Macnaughton, L.S. et al. (2016) The response of muscle protein synthesis following whole-body resistance exercise is greater following 40 g than 20 g of ingested whey protein, *Physiological Reports*, 4(15), p.e12893.

Mantantzis, K. et al. (2019) Sugar rush or sugar crash? A meta-analysis of carbohydrate effects on mood, *Neuroscience & Biobehavioral Reviews*, 101, pp.45–67.

Margolis, K.G., Cryan, J.F. and Mayer, E.A. (2021) The microbiota-gut-brain axis: From motility to mood, *Gastroenterology* (New York, 1943), 160(5), pp.1486–1501. doi:10.1053/j.gastro.2020.10.066.

McAlindon, T.E. et al. (2011) Change in knee osteoarthritis cartilage detected by delayed gadolinium enhanced magnetic resonance imaging following treatment with collagen hydrolysate: A pilot randomized controlled trial, *Osteoarthritis and Cartilage*, 19(4), pp.399–405.

Molaeikhaletabadi, M. et al. (2022) Short-term effects of low-fat chocolate milk on delayed onset muscle soreness and performance in players on a women's university badminton team, *International Journal of Environmental Research and Public Health*, 19(6), p.3677.

Mountjoy, M. *et al.* (2014) The IOC consensus statement: Beyond the female athlete triad—relative energy deficiency in sport (RED-S), *British Journal of Sports Medicine,* 48(7), pp.491–497.

Mountjoy, M. et al. (2018) International Olympic Committee (IOC) consensus statement on relative energy deficiency in sport (RED-S): 2018 update, *International Journal of Sport Nutrition and Exercise Metabolism*, 28(4), pp.316–331.

NDA, E.S.P. (2015) Scientific opinion on the safety of caffeine, *Efsa Journal*, 13(5), p.4102.

Owens, D.J. et al. (2019) Exercise-induced muscle damage: What is it, what causes it and what are the nutritional solutions? *European Journal of Sport Science*, 19(1), pp.71–85.

Palacios, C. (2006) The role of nutrients in bone health, from A to Z, *Critical Reviews in Food Science and Nutrition*, 46(8), pp.621–628.

Passeron, T. et al. (2019) Sunscreen photoprotection and vitamin D status, *British Journal of Dermatology*, 181(5), pp.916–931.

Pouresmaeili, F. et al. (2018) A comprehensive overview on osteoporosis and its risk factors, *Therapeutics and Clinical Risk Management*, 14, p.2029.

Shaw, G. et al. (2017) Vitamin c–enriched gelatin supplementation before intermittent activity augments collagen synthesis, *The American Journal of Clinical Nutrition*, 105(1), pp.136–143.

Smith, A. (2002) Effects of caffeine on human behavior, *Food and Chemical Toxicology*, 40(9), pp.1243–1255.

Smith-Ryan, A.E. et al. (2020) Nutritional considerations and strategies to facilitate injury recovery and rehabilitation, *Journal of Athletic Training*, 55(9), pp.918–930.

Trangmar, S.J. and González-Alonso, J. (2017) New insights into the impact of dehydration on blood flow and metabolism during exercise, *Exercise and Sport Sciences Reviews*, 45(3), pp.146–153.

Tucker, T. (2006) *The great starvation experiment: The heroic men who starved so that millions could live.* Simon and Schuster, New York, pp.128–162.

Williams, N.C. et al. (2019) Immune nutrition and exercise: Narrative review and practical recommendations, *European Journal of Sport Science*, 19(1), pp.49–61.

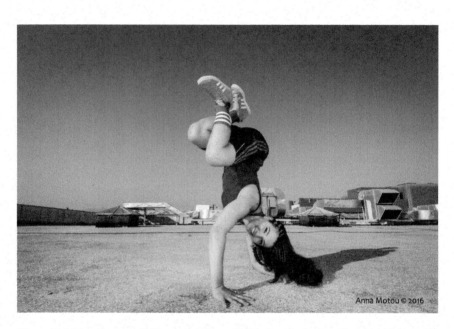

Photo 12.1 Dancers can follow partially or fully plant-based meal plans: Chapter 12 discusses how dancers meet their nutritional needs when using mainly, or only, plant-based foods.

Source: Credit: Photo courtesy of Anna Moutou

12 Plant-based diets for dancers

Contents

I Introduction to plant-based diets for dancers

Human beings around the world, including of course dancers, eat and enjoy a wide range of plant foods; fruits and vegetables, including starchy vegetables such as potatoes and sweet potatoes; nuts and seeds; beans and lentils; and grains. Many grains are used around the world, often as the basis of meals, whether transformed into products such as pasta, couscous, noodles or bread, or with more minimal processing, enough to make them edible such as rice, oats and maize. Rice must be milled even to produce wholegrain brown rice while oats need to be cleaned to remove inedible hulls as a minimum. Maize needs little processing to be eaten as sweetcorn, but considerably more to produce maize flour, corn oil or corn syrup. Nuts and seeds can be the source of oils and spreads to combine with other, often plant based, foods as well as eaten in their original form.

A plant-based diet does not have to mean a plant-only diet, although it can do. 'Plant-based' can mean anything from a completely vegan diet which contains no products of animal origin, to a diet where meals include some animal foods such as meat, poultry, fish, eggs or dairy products. When animal foods are included, they will be in smaller proportions than typically

DOI: 10.4324/9781003219002-12

seen, with more emphasis on foods derived from plants – fruits and vegetables, wholegrains, pulses, nuts, seeds and oils. There are a number of reasons why a dancer may choose to opt for a plant-based diet, each of which will impact on their nutrition. Reasons might include:

- To reduce their 'carbon footprint' and eat a more sustainable diet, that is better for the future of the planet. Your carbon footprint is the amount of carbon dioxide your lifestyle produces. Diet is an important component of this, but it is not the only factor and is often not straightforward. Depending on whether a food has needed transporting, and if so, the type of transport will make a substantial difference. Sustainable diets are explored in Section IV.
- Because they don't wish to eat food that involves animals being killed.
- Because they are concerned about the way animal farming is undertaken.
- To spend less money on food: we will explore ways to eat economically whether fully plant based or not.
- Because they believe it will help their health and dance performance.
- For religious reasons: most religions have some food rules, some ask that followers are completely vegetarian.

Including a number of different plant-based foods daily is a strategy that results in a wide range of macro-, micro- and phytonutrients being consumed. Aiming for 30 different types of plants per week, i.e., fruit/veg/salad/grain/pulses, using seasonal options where possible is a target that may help the gut microbiome (Lee et al., 2020).

The next section explores the practicalities of a vegetarian diet and is aimed at all dancers, as most, if not all, dancers will eat at least one cooked meal each day and may have one or more days when they are vegetarian whether by choice or due to circumstances such as finances or skills. Vegetarian sources of protein can be cheaper than meat or fish, and some dancers prefer not to have to prepare meat or fish meals, others may find some enjoyable vegetarian meals that are easier and quicker to prepare than meat or fish dishes.

II Vegetarian diets for dancers

The main three subdivisions of vegetarian diets are:

A   Lacto-ovo vegetarians. Meat, poultry and fish are excluded, but eggs and dairy products are included. This will mean that milk, cheese and yoghurt will be included which could be from cows' milk or equally goats' milk or sheeps' milk.
B   Lacto vegetarians: meat, poultry, fish and eggs are avoided, while dairy products are included.
C   Ovo vegetarians: meat, poultry, fish and dairy products are avoided, but eggs and egg products are included.

Dancers who describe themselves as 'flexitarian' are generally vegetarians most of the time, but who will occasionally include meat, fish or other non-vegetarian items.

There are a further group: pescatarians, who are those who include fish but not meat or poultry. Pescatarians are not vegetarians but do sometimes get classed with vegetarians. Pescatarian is a relatively new term from the 1990s, now widely accepted. There is sometimes confusion amongst caterers as to whether vegetarians do eat fish. If you are pescatarian or vegetarian, we would advise you to be as specific as possible as to which group you fall into to ensure you are able to access suitable foods when away from home.

The smaller the range of foods that is eaten, the more there needs to be a focus to ensure all nutrients are covered. Vegetarians including eggs and dairy products do need to be mindful with regard to some nutrient requirements, in particular protein and iron, during a dance career but face fewer challenges than those who exclude either dairy or eggs or vegans.

Planning a vegetarian diet for dance/how do I best plan a healthy vegetarian diet?

A great starting point is to remember that variety is really helpful in achieving good nutrition. No single food, or even two or three foods can supply all the nutrients that we need. The more variety you include the more you are likely to get a good intake of nutrients – and the food is more interesting! A diet with a high proportion of plant foods is likely to be bulky, and those with smaller appetites, or who find it difficult to eat large volumes of food before dance will need to carefully consider how they meet their energy requirements and not compromise their health due to early fullness from the high fibre plant foods that then mean enough food isn't eaten (Melin et al., 2016).

Breakfast

Breakfast is a key time to deliver nutrients that will fuel the dancer's day from around mid-morning to mid-afternoon, depending on food choices. Many breakfasts are naturally vegetarian, including the oat-based staples of porridge/muesli/granola that work well for many dancers. If you aren't using cow's milk/yoghurt (or sheep/goat equivalents) in/on porridge/oat-based cereal, do check that any plant alternative is delivering some useful nutrients. Milk is an excellent source of protein, calcium and iodine, as well as a significant amount of protein. These nutrients and alternative sources are covered in the vegan section below.

An alternative to porridge or cereal is including eggs with breakfast. The nutritional content is similar whether boiled, poached or fried with minimal oil. Scrambled eggs for training/performance days are best made with minimal added fats so as not to slow digestion down when you have a demanding day ahead. Serve with toast/a muffin or bagel or any locally available carb choice that tastes good. Use whole eggs for the best range of nutrients. For those who are not including eggs, then scrambled tofu is a useful option at breakfast. Adding some vegetables, whether tomatoes, mushrooms or something green, will add useful vitamins and minerals whether using tofu or eggs. If using eggs but time is a challenge, then cooking several eggs at a times and using them over the next few days (maximum a week, in a fridge) can work well. When time allows 'French toast' ('eggy bread') is another way to serve eggs – just watch the oil content or digestion may be slowed down.

Cottage cheese or another lower-fat cheese can make a change for breakfast – with all of the protein suggestions remember to plan in variety.

Cereal can be a good option if served with some fruit and maybe a few nuts or seeds to add protein, vitamins and minerals. Be cautious in your choices – highly processed cereals are less likely to keep you full for long and often deliver less nutrients overall, so they are best kept for occasional use at times when this isn't a problem. Oats in muesli or granola are a good option, check the ingredients list to find one which is lower rather than higher in sugar, or better still check out recipes and devise your own. If you really struggle to eat breakfast, then a bowl of a cereal you can tolerate, with some milk/yoghurt and any additions of fruit and nuts/seeds you can manage is going to provide a better start to the day then nothing.

Lunches and dinners/mid-day and evening meals

There is a pitfall with main meals that it's best to avoid: sometimes dancers, particularly vegetarians, who are short of time end up with many meals each week where cheese is the main source of protein, as it is relatively inexpensive and needs no preparation. While cheese can help you meet your protein needs, depending on the meals chosen, the portions needed may push your fat intake up, which can compromise your carb intake. Also, cheese is a great source of calcium, but contains almost no iron, so a diet with much of the protein being from cheese will be at risk of being low in iron. As iron intakes are a concern for dancers, it makes sense to include a wide variety of vegetarian protein sources. For the advantages of different protein sources, see Chapter 5.

A healthy vegetarian diet for dancers requires planning. Time spent on planning out lunches and dinners for a week, or having two to three weeks that can be rotated, is well worth it.

As you saw in Chapter 5, different foods supply different proportions of EAAs (essential amino acids). Planning meals that naturally optimise the balance of amino acids is a constructive way to support your nutritional intake. Some examples that give a great range of amino acids and combine meals with lower protein content with meals with higher protein content are:

1 Lunch: Wheat tortilla with mixed beans, salad, grated cheese and gua-camole; fruit and yoghurt.
   Dinner: Omelette with new potatoes and vegetables, slice of banana bread.
2 Lunch: Lentil and vegetable curry with rice and plain yoghurt.
   Dinner: Quorn or soya mince bolognaise with pasta and side salad.
   Lentils or beans, which are low in EAA methionine, are combined with rice or wheat which are low in EAAs lysine and threonine, so combining these foods results in potentially more useable protein. The profiles of Quorn and soya are excellent, and there is no need to combine another food from a protein point of view.

III Vegan diets

A vegan diet is one that included no products of animal origin. Vegans exclude meat, fish, eggs and all dairy products. This usually includes no foods containing even small amounts of animal products. Some vegans also exclude honey. While it is possible to achieve a vegan diet that will meet a dancer's needs, this requires planning, and consideration of which supplements is necessary, as a vegan diet does not contain adequate vitamin B12 unless fortified foods or supplements are included. Iodine, calcium and iron are other minerals of concern which will be explored shortly.

Protein historically has been a challenge for vegans, as although there are plant-based foods with fair or good amounts of protein, the range of foods has been narrow. Beans and lentils are relatively bulky, as the equivalent to a small portion of meat/fish/three eggs is a 400g can of beans or lentils! Tofu is less bulky, and often a good option, but some people find it less palatable unless prepared creatively. Soya mince is useful and versatile, but a vegan diet can be overly reliant on soy if care is not taken. Some Quorn products are vegan, and there are also new products such as meat alternatives that use protein options such as pea protein. Nuts and seeds are good sources of protein on a weight-for-weight basis, but their high-fat content limits their use as the only protein in a meal. One option is to combine nuts or seeds with low-fat pulses, for example, using both beans and nuts in a risotto, adding nuts to a lentil curry. Serving with grains, such as pasta, couscous or rice will provide some additional protein.

If you are considering a vegan diet but are a picky eater, and not keen on many of the vegan protein options, then it would be good to get some professional advice from a qualified dance dietitian to work out how you will meet your needs.

Vitamin B12

Vitamin B12 is not found in significant amounts in plant products. For more details on the role of vitamin B12 in human health, see Appendix A. Vegans

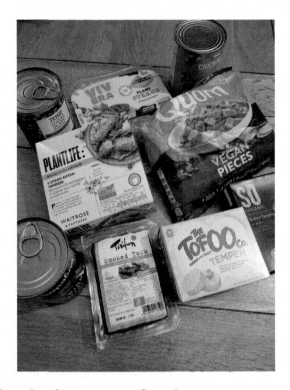

Photo 12.2 Examples of vegan sources of protein.

need to include a supplement to avoid long-term problems with the nervous system and a particular type of anaemia where the red blood cells are too large and too few.

Iodine

For non-vegans iodine, needed for normal metabolism, is usually obtained from dairy foods and fish, especially white fish. In some countries, iodine is routinely added to salt, but this is not the case in the UK at the time of writing. Even in the UK, it is possible to buy iodised salt, but many dancers use limited amounts of salt, so this is not a realistic solution to meeting requirements for many. Seaweed and seaweed products can contain very large amounts of iodine. Although vegans can obtain iodine from seaweed, because amounts are not consistent, and can be very high, relying on seaweed is not generally recommended. There are inexpensive supplements available that contain B12, iodine as well as vitamin D in formats suitable for vegans. Some plant-based milk alternatives are fortified with iodine, and these are recommended for any dancer not using dairy products.

Iron

Plant-based iron is less well absorbed than the iron from animal products. Male dancers meeting their energy and protein needs with a variety of foods are likely to be able to meet their iron needs, and female dancers on higher intake days, as shown in Table 12.1. This day has been planned to include a number of iron-rich foods such as the bean chilli.

Calcium

Typically in omnivorous diets, a high proportion of calcium is derived from dairy milk, cheese and yoghurt. In a vegan diet, plant-based milk alternatives contain very variable amounts of calcium: many are fortified, but not all, and

Table 12.1 Iron content of a sample vegan menu for a male dancer, low intensity dance day or a female dancer moderate to higher intensity dance day

Examples of iron from vegan foods

Food and portion	Iron content (mg)
Oats for porridge, 60 g	2.2
Soya milk, 400 ml	1.7
1 tbsp peanut butter	0.3
Medium banana	0.3
Four large slices wholemeal bread	3.6
Houmous : 60 g (4 tbsps)	1.1
Quorn 70 g	0.4
Salad for sandwich – good portion, 60 g	0.2
Cereal bar, average	1.1
Malt loaf	0.6
Bean chilli	4.3
Brown rice 80 g uncooked (½ mug)	1.0
Broccoli, 100 g steamed	0.8
Soya yoghurt, fortified 150 g	0.7
Mixed nuts 60 g	1.8
Muesli 60 g	1.6
Total	21.7

Around 9–11 mg/day iron is accepted as enough to meet the requirements of most men from age 18. Around 15–18 mg iron/day is accepted as enough to meet the requirements of most women from the age of 15 until the menopause	Iron from plant sources is less well absorbed than from animal sources. Having vitamin C from fruit/veg with a meal will help absorption, while drinking tea or coffee with, or soon after a plant-based meal can reduce iron absorption by at least 40–50%

Table 12.2 Sources of calcium in a vegan diet

Vegan sources of calcium	
Food and portion	Calcium content (mg)
Fortified plant 'milk' alternative: 100 ml	120+ (check labelling)
Tofu: 100 g: higher value is for calcium set tofu Soy and edamame beans are also a useful source	175–350
Sesame seeds: 10 g. Many other seeds are also a useful source of calcium	67
Broccoli, steamed: 100 g	44
Orange average	38
Soya yoghurt, fruit, fortified: 100 g	120 (check labelling)
Kidney beans: 100 g cooked/canned (drained)	71
Wholemeal bread one medium slice	40
Oats, unfortified: 50 g	25
Brazil nuts: 30 g. Almonds are also a useful source	51
Kale, cooked: 100 g	150
Dancers from the age of 18 years are advised to aim for at least 700 mg calcium daily	

those making their own alternatives perhaps from oats or nuts will need to be particularly mindful of calcium sources in their diet. Table 12.2 shows the calcium content of some vegan foods with at least a reasonable calcium content. Many other foods will provide smaller amounts that nonetheless can help you reach an adequate intake of calcium.

Vitamin D

There are very few foods which naturally provide vitamin D, and the only vegan option would be mushrooms exposed to sunshine in the middle of the day for at least 15 minutes.

There are a number of foods which are fortified with vitamin D including milk alternatives and many breakfast cereals. Vegan dancers are advised to follow the same advice as for all dancers on taking a supplement at least through winter months; see Chapter 8 for more information.

Planning a vegan diet that meets dancers' requirements

Including the widest range of foods possible will make achieving a vegan diet that meets dance requirements the best it can be. This is best done by planning meals and snacks for at least a day at a time, to allow variety in proteins in particular, as well as including adequate carbohydrates and fats. Be aware that there are some products that are marketed as plant alternatives to meat that are very poor substitutes, and not protein sources. These include jackfruit, banana blossom, and types of vegan 'cheese' that are in fact just fat and starch. These can of course be included in meals for flavour or texture, but one or more sources of plant protein will be needed as well.

Vegan protein: challenges to nutritional availability

Plant proteins often contain anti-nutritional factors, which are compounds that can reduce the digestibility of the protein. These compounds include trypsin inhibitors, tannins and phytates which each work in different ways. Trypsin inhibitors in beans, lentils and grains block the action of trypsin, a digestive enzyme involved with breaking down protein. Tannins, found in some grains, beans and peas, are thought to reduce the digestibility of carbohydrates, minerals and protein by inhibiting digestive enzymes. Phytate, found in nuts, seeds and grains, binds with proteins in the digestive tract, reducing their absorption.

Making vegan proteins more available

Preparation techniques can mitigate the effect of the anti-nutritional factors. For example, soaking, fermentation and germination all can reduce levels of phytate in foods (Lynch et al., 2018). Those relying on plant proteins exclusively may benefit from aiming above the 1.6 g/kg body weight advised in Chapter 5.

Vegan Nutrient Challenges

Nutrient at risk	Nutrient needed for	Options to consider
Vitamin B12	Production of normal red blood cells	Supplement or fortified foods to supply 1.5–4 mcg daily
Iodine	Normal metabolism	Supplement or fortified foods to supply 140–150 mcg daily
Vitamin D	Calcium absorption and many other roles	Supplement or fortified foods to supply 10–25 mcg daily
Iron	Red blood cells to transport oxygen	Good portions of beans and lentils regularly
Zinc	Enzyme synthesis, regulate mood, immune system, wound healing	Wheatgerm, seeds, nuts, wholegrains. Green veg provide moderate amounts
Calcium	Bone health, muscle contraction, nerve impulse conduction	Use fortified plant based alternatives to milk and yoghurt

IV Sustainable eating

Sustainable eating is the concept of meeting your nutritional needs safely without negatively impacting on the environment. It focuses on choices of food which have a reduced carbon footprint compared with a typical dancer's diet. The concept can apply to all dancers, not just those who are completely plant based in their food choices. It covers the impact of agriculture on land use, the need to protect biodiversity, ecosystems and natural resources, including how fishing impacts the oceans and also how food production impacts the production of gases which contribute to global warming (World Health Organization, 2019). Many dancers are concerned about global warming and keen to minimise their personal impact on this. This is an important part of sustainable eating, but there are additional areas which impact more widely on society which are worth exploring briefly. Sustainable eating is relevant whether you are completely plant based in your food choices or include foods of animal origin.

The 'carbon footprint' of the food you eat is the term often used when thinking about sustainable eating. The carbon footprint of a food is the volume of greenhouse gases produced in growing, processing, packaging, distribution, storage and cooking that food. A 'greenhouse gas' is a gas in the earth's atmosphere that traps heat and contributes to global warming.

Greenhouse gases include carbon dioxide, methane, nitrous oxide and industrial gases containing fluorine. Although not all greenhouse gases contain carbon, the terms greenhouse gas and carbon footprint tend to be used interchangeably. While carbon dioxide is the primary greenhouse gas, around 75–80%, compared with around 10–15% from methane, the methane is estimated to have over 20 times the impact on global warming compared with carbon dioxide.

The second area of sustainable eating is food security, which focuses more at a population level, aiming to ensure everyone has at the minimum amount of nutrients to meet basic requirements. It is relevant to the dancer though, as it is important that reductions in carbon footprint don't result in a diet that is no longer nutritionally fit for purpose for the dancer.

The third area of sustainable diets looks at public health goals: which foods should be increased/reduced to improve the population's health (Springmann et al., 2018).

Reducing your carbon footprint without losing out on nutrition

- Buying locally produced produce is one way that can often reduce your carbon footprint and has little impact on nutrition, depending on the food.
- Where a food isn't produced locally, for example, exotic fruit and some nuts, the further the food has travelled the greater the additional greenhouse gas production before the food is consumed. This does need to

be weighed against the increases in greenhouse gas production from heated greenhouses being used to produce food locally.

- The lowest greenhouse gas option will be to buy local, seasonal fruits and vegetables that are grown outdoors or in a greenhouse heated just by sun: make sure you know what's in season for your area when shopping.
- You minimise your carbon footprint with regard to packaging if you try to buy products that are packaged as little as possible. One important area is the use of bottled water. Use tap water where possible – bottled water has a carbon footprint around 300 times greater than tap water (Botto, 2009).

The relative carbon footprint of different farming methods is more complex and needs consideration of whether land use has changed, such as where forests have been removed so that crops can be grown. Dancers interested in this area are encouraged to research this area further; it is beyond the scope of this book to explore all the factors that need to be considered in weighing up the carbon cost of growing specific foods under different conditions.

Food storage does have an impact on the carbon footprint of a food if refrigeration is required, but this also reduces food spoilage and potentially wastage.

Reducing food waste

Reducing food waste is a vital part of minimising your carbon footprint. This can be a real challenge for many dancers, as unexpected changes to schedule can affect all dancers, including students, professionals and teachers. Avoiding food waste does require thought and planning.

Tips to reduce food waste:

1 Plan meals for several days in advance and shop for those meals. At busy times think about meals for which, if plans change, the ingredients can be frozen as long as they are within use by dates.
2 Try and buy amounts that are useable rather than bigger packs that may seem to be better value, but will only save you money if the whole pack is used.
3 Fruit can be frozen for use in a dessert or smoothie – some fruits such as berries and apples may be better if pureed before freezing.
4 Use frozen vegetables at busy times – they are as nutritious as fresh.
5 Keep an eye on 'use by' dates for foods in the fridge – if possible put new food at the back of each shelf and move older food to the front so it doesn't get overlooked. Is there a way to cook the item and then freeze it, if it can't be frozen as bought?

6 Keep an eye on your fridge temperature: it may need to be adjusted if the air temperature changes, and according to how full it is.

7 Liaise with peers if you can only buy perishable foods in large amounts; for example, seasonal fruits and vegetables – can you share a large amount with several other dancers?

8 Bread and bread products can be frozen in practical amounts, for example, two to four slices of bread and one to two bagels.

9 Think about the right portion sizes for you – minimise plate waste as best as you can. Serve yourself the portion you think works initially, if you have possibly cooked a bit too much: you can always have a second helping – or use leftovers towards a meal for the next day.

10 If you can, either compost inedible food waste, or use local composting schemes.

11 Check out websites/social media for more advice/suggestions on this area.

12 Think about food storage and transport – use containers which can be re-used/recycled as far as possible.

Dancers and athletes are advised to have a higher intake of protein to ensure they meet their requirements to benefit from training and perform at their best. Good sources of protein tend to be foods which have a higher carbon footprint, though this can depend on other factors such as transport

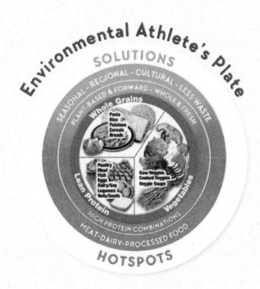

Figure 12.1 The Environmental impact of the Athletes Plate food model.

and processing. Research has begun looking at the environmental impact of a widely used tool in sports nutrition, The Athletes Plate (Reguant-Closa et al., 2019). There is a version looking at the environmental impact of the higher protein recommendations for sport, which is shown in Figure 12.1 (Reguant-Closer et al., 2020, reproduced under the Creative Commons International Public License – Attribution 4.0 International – CC BY 4.0).

This plate model identifies the areas of the traditional athlete plate model that, while providing sound advice to athletes on nutrition, does not address the impact of this on the environment.

The authors suggest that meeting the increased demands for activity while minimising the impact on the environment is best done by:

1 Fuelling the work being done – meeting targets for all macronutrients and not overly relying on protein.
2 Using proteins with a lower carbon footprint by replacing some animal protein with plant protein, and within the animal protein fraction, prioritise milk, eggs, poultry and pork over ruminant meat and cheese. Checking sources of any protein supplements used to make sure they result in minimal food waste.
3 Using fresh, seasonal, regional and unprocessed foods.
4 Limiting frozen and canned products.

Sustainable sources of protein

Beef has a higher carbon footprint than lamb while pork, game meats, chicken and eggs have a much lower carbon footprint than lamb. The carbon footprint of beef will however depend on whether the beef has been grazing on grass or fed with grains or other foods specifically grown for the cattle. Grazing cattle on land that is not suitable for growing other crops is more sustainable than using land that could support crops to be consumed by humans. Opting for beef reared more sustainably together with using smaller amounts of meat combined with beans and lentils, such as chilli con carne, or beef and bean burritos allows a reduced carbon footprint within a diet that isn't too bulky and provides good quality protein combined with vitamins and minerals that are less available in a completely plant-based diet.

Fish or shellfish need to be caught or produced in a way that allows stocks to replenish and that does not cause unnecessary damage to marine animals and plants.

To ensure there are enough fish and shellfish to eat in the longer term, choose from as wide a range of these foods as possible. Eating a limited range of fish results in the numbers of these fish falling very low, due to overfishing of these stocks. Overfishing endangers the future supply of the fish and can also cause damage to the environment from which the fish is caught. Choosing sardines, herring and molluscs (clams, scallops, cockles, oysters, cuttlefish and squid) rather than other fish/seafood can usefully reduce your carbon footprint.

Although dairy milk, yoghurt and cheese have a higher carbon footprint than plant alternatives, it is important to be mindful of the nutrition the plant-based options supply. While there are some useful alternatives emerging onto the market, that have comparable nutrition to the dairy versions, there are also a number of low-nutrient alternatives, such as some vegan alternatives to cheese that are just starch and oil with some added vitamins/minerals, and some nut containing alternatives to milk which have a very low nut content. The resources required for manufacturing, packaging and transport may not offer a useful alternative when looking at the provision of nutrients. Checking the protein content on labelling and comparing to conventional options is a useful way to identify the best options.

There are a number of mycoprotein products available, the most widely known is Quorn. Quorn is comparable with pork and poultry for greenhouse gas production but uses less water and land and is a good option as a protein source (Souza Filho et al., 2019). Beans and lentils are the most sustainable sources of protein, and including regularly in your diet is a great option.

Nuts and seeds have a higher carbon footprint than beans and lentils, but still lower than most fish and all meat products.

Opting for vegan meals at two meals per day is a practical way for non-vegans to make choices that reduce their carbon footprint substantially but without opting for a fully vegan diet.

Sustainable sources of carbohydrates

Carbohydrate refuelling after demanding dance training or performance is best begun as quickly as possible. Recovery also requires repair, which involves timely ingestion of protein. Rest and rehydration are the final two aspects of recovery. Taking note of the best timings for nutrition intake will allow dancers to benefit physiologically from hard training and performances while also minimising the impact on the planet. See Chapters 4 and 5 for more information on this.

Sustainable sources of fats

Production of olive oil has been estimated to result in the removal of carbon dioxide from the atmosphere rather than any additional contribution (Proietti at al., 2017). Olive oil isn't suitable for all uses, but the combination of unsaturated fats and negative carbon footprint makes it a good choice, where it can be used. Tree nuts have a slightly lower carbon footprint than seeds, but this would not outweigh the advantages of cooking with an oil suitable for the purpose required. Butter does have a significantly higher carbon footprint, so environmentally is best used sparingly. A further aspect of oils is the container they are sold in, and trying to ensure this can be recycled as far as possible.

V Organic food

Food grown organically is grown without the use of synthetic chemicals, such as manufactured pesticides, including weed killers and fertilisers, and doesn't contain genetically modified organisms (GMOs). Naturally derived pesticides such as citronella and clove oil are permitted under some circumstances (UK Soil Association)

Crop rotation is practiced, where fields are used for different crops in different years, which can help maintain fertile soil, along with the use of compost and animal manure.

Animals raised organically will not have received antibiotics routinely. Animal welfare is an important part of organic farming including the animals' living conditions and feed, their transportation and humane slaughter. Organically raised animals will have more living space than those reared non-organically.

The differences in the way soil and produce are kept healthy and how animals are reared has an impact on the cost of organic food.

Organic food choices and budget challenges

The amount of money dancers have available to spend on food is often limited. This can bring some very difficult challenges and decisions about the best choices when food shopping. Information about the nutrient content of organic produce suggests that some fruits and vegetables may be higher in antioxidants compared to non-organic versions; however, this is not consistent, and the difference in price may well make the relative cost of those nutrients greater, even if the content is higher than in the conventional varieties. There are many factors involved, particularly with fruit and vegetables, as storage can make a big difference to the content of some nutrients, with the freshest options being the best choice.

When money is limited, and choices have to be made about whether to buy organic produce or not, the priority is to get all the nutrients you need. If buying organic produce will compromise being able to have at least five portions of fruits and vegetables daily, or will compromise your intake of macronutrients then you are best to buy conventional versions of food to meet your requirements and include a good variety of fruit and vegetables.

VI Phytochemicals and their benefits for health and performance

Phytochemicals/phytonutrients

Phytochemicals are often known as phytonutrients. This term is more relatable to nutrition so will be used here. Phytonutrients are substances found in certain plants which are believed to be beneficial to human health and help prevent various diseases when sufficient quantities are consumed. There are many thousands of phytonutrients found in fruits, vegetables, grains, beans, nuts and seeds.

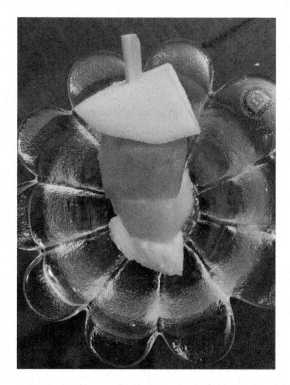

Photo 12.3 Fruit is a great source of phytochemicals.

Perhaps the best known phytonutrients are those found in fruits, particularly in cherries and berries, but vegetables as well as other plant foods, such as legumes (beans and lentils) and grains can supply us with phytonutrients. The effects of phytonutrients when used as supplements are looked at in Chapter 8.

Phytochemicals can be divided into groups according to their chemical structure. The main group is polyphenols, but there are useful phytonutrients in the remaining groups which are the terpenoids, alkaloids, phytosterols and organosulphur compounds. Over 8,000 polyphenols have been identified so far. Table 12.3 shows information on some of the most relevant phytonutrients for dancers.

A note about phytoestrogens

Phytoestrogens have a similar structure to oestrogen and there has been much debate over recent years about what, if any, are the effects of soy included regularly in the diet. A review concluded that there are both advantages and disadvantages, but moderate intakes of soy are unlikely to cause harm. Asian populations do consume soy regularly over their lives

Table 12.3 Relevant phytonutrients for dancers

Phytonutrient group and name	Food sources for the phytonutrient	Purpose of phytonutrient
Polyphenols: flavonoids – over 4,000 individual compounds	Fruits, vegetables, cereals, drinks such as tea and coffee NB: Apples, pears, grapes cherries and berries have particularly high levels of useful polyphenols	Most work as antioxidants and are anti-inflammatory. Some have an anti-cancer effect. Tart cherry juice has been used specifically in both sport and dance to minimise exercise-induced muscle damage and accelerate recovery from muscle damage. These properties are thought to be due to the high levels of polyphenols (Brown et al., 2019)
Polyphenols: flavonoids: isoflavones	Soy	Act as phytoestrogens: Some isoflavones are absorbed by the body, while microbes in the gut break others down into either oestrogen-like compounds or anti-oestrogenic compounds with opposite effects
Polyphenols: tannins	Tea is a rich source, also some fruits and seeds, with lower levels in a range of plant foods	Antimicrobial effects. Conflicting evidence about their impact on risks of cancers and on reducing nutrient availability, for example, iron
Terpenoids: carotenes: 40 yellow, orange and red compounds	Orange, yellow and red foods, such as carrots, melon, also some dark green leafy vegetables	Anti-oxidants, can support the immune system, may help bone density and can help prevent some types of eye problems
Terpenoids: d-limonene	Citrus fruit	Protective effects against cancer and diabetes; anti-oxidant and anti-inflammatory properties
Alkaloids: theobromine	Cocoa and chocolate, and in smaller amounts in tea	Can be used to make caffeine. Theobromine can help with alertness and mood in appropriate amounts
Phytosterols: B-sitosterol	Good sources include avocado, soybeans, some nuts, some vegetable oils and some grains, many other plant foods have smaller amounts	Anti-inflammatory, cholesterol lowering effects and possibly also benefits for wound healing, anti-oxidant prevention of cell damage and reduce cancer risks
Organosulphur compounds: isothiocyanates	Cruciferous vegetables such as broccoli, cabbage, cauliflower Bok choi, Brussels sprouts, turnip, radish, swede (rutabaga) and watercress	Help protect against cancer
Organosulphur compounds: allyl sulphur compounds	Garlic	Help protect against heart disease

with no obvious consequences and using foods rather than products supplemented with soy is likely to be the best option for health benefits from soy (Patisaul & Jefferson, 2010).

With the wide range of beneficial phytochemical found in plant-based foods, all dancers are encouraged to include a wide variety of plant-based foods both day to day and week to week to get maximum benefit. Ongoing research over the next few years will bring more clarity to this area, and looking out for updates is a good plan.

VII Resources

Vegetarian/Vegan Athlete's Plate® | Sustainability, Wellness & Learning (SWELL) (uccs.edu).
Carbon footprint calculator, e.g., WWF Footprint Calculator.

VIII Learning outcomes

After reading this chapter the reader should be able to:

1   Explain different types of vegetarian diets and how these differ from a vegan diet.
2   Review the nutrients that can be lacking in a highly/exclusively plant-based diets and options to improve intakes.
3   Discuss the aspects of food sourcing that impact sustainability.
4   State examples of phytonutrients, foods they are found in and potential benefits to dancers.

References

Botto, S. (2009) Tap water vs. bottled water in a footprint integrated approach, *Nature Preceedings*, 7th July, pp.1.

Brown, M.A., Stevenson, E.J. and Howatson, G. (2019) Montmorency tart cherry (*Prunus cerasus L.*) supplementation accelerates recovery from exercise-induced muscle damage in females, *European Journal of Sport Science*, 19(1), pp.95–102.

Lee, K.A. et al. (2020) Role of the gut microbiome for cancer patients receiving immunotherapy: Dietary and treatment implications, *European Journal of Cancer*, 138, pp.149–155.

Lynch, H., Johnston, C. and Wharton, C. (2018) Plant-based diets: Considerations for environmental impact, protein quality, and exercise performance, *Nutrients,* 10(12), pp.1841.

Melin, A. et al. (2016) Low-energy density and high fiber intake are dietary concerns in female endurance athletes, *Scandinavian Journal of Medicine & Science in Sports*, 26(9), pp.1060–1071.

Patisaul, H.B. and Jefferson, W. (2010) The pros and cons of phytoestrogens, *Frontiers in Neuroendocrinology*, 31(4), pp.400–419.

Proietti, S. et al. (2017) Extra virgin olive oil as carbon negative product: Experimental analysis and validation of results, *Journal of Cleaner Production*, 166, pp.550–562.

Reguant-Closa, A. et al. (2019) Validation of the athlete's plate nutrition educational tool: Phase I, *International Journal of Sport Nutrition and Exercise Metabolism*, 29(6), pp.628–635.

Reguant-Closa, A. et al. (2020) The environmental impact of the athlete's plate nutrition education tool, *Nutrients*, 12(8), p.2484.

Souza Filho, P.F. et al. (2019) Mycoprotein: Environmental impact and health aspects, *World Journal of Microbiology and Biotechnology*, 35(10), pp.1–8.

Springmann, M. et al. (2018) Health and nutritional aspects of sustainable diet strategies and their association with environmental impacts: A global modelling analysis with country-level detail, *The Lancet Planetary Health*, 2(10), pp.e451–e461.

World Health Organization (2019) *Sustainable healthy diets: Guiding principles*, Food & Agriculture Org.

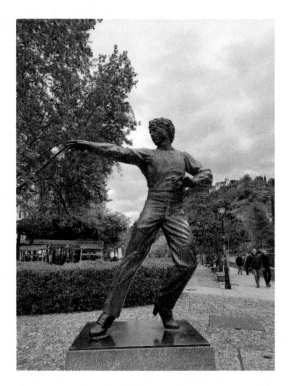

Photo 13.1 **All human bodies have their challenges: longevity as a dancer is helped by taking care of your body, including dietary changes where necessary.**
Credit: Jasmine Challis

13 Clinical nutrition

Contents

I Introduction

Nutrition can make a huge difference not just to performance but also in the management of a number of medical conditions – and of course, dancers are not exempt from having medical conditions that can require and benefit from dietary modifications. This makes life more complicated for sure – trying to combine the recommendations for a medical condition – or even more than one medical condition – with performance recommendations is a challenge.

If you are in this position then if at all possible you will do best to get individualised advice from a registered dietitian who has an understanding of both dance and your medical condition. If this isn't possible then there are a couple of other options that may help you. Dietitians are used to communicating – so it may be best for your clinical dietitian to liaise with a dance/sports dietitian to work out how best to combine the requirements for both. This would be useful in more unusual conditions such as PKU, cystic fibrosis, Crohn's disease or epilepsy treated with a ketogenic diet.

DOI: 10.4324/9781003219002-13

Otherwise, your clinical dietitian may be able to tailor your advice using the information in this book.

Due to limitations of space, this chapter is focussing on five areas of health that are more likely to be of relevance to dancers and where nutrition is important in management.

II Gut health and immunity

Your gut is a main gateway from the environment around you, with the infection risks it can bring, into your body. The topic of gut health: the balance of microorganisms, in particular bacteria, in your intestines, and their location – is a relatively new aspect of human, and dancer, health. Not only can the variety and amounts of the different bacteria impact health, in particular, they can impact the immune system (Morgan & Huttenhower, 2012).

The combined genetic material of the microorganisms in the gut is known as the microbiome, and the microbiota is the name given to the collection of microorganisms you have in your gut.

This is a relatively new area of health, and it is likely that research will identify more information about our microbiome and health and performance over the next few years.

It is already known that your gut microbiota can influence many areas of your health from innate immunity to appetite regulation and energy metabolism. It is also well established that the presence of your gut microbiota enables you to use food as efficiently as possible: the energy stored in some types of fibre can be salvaged by some bacteria, with the production of short-chain fatty acids (SCFA) which can then be used by the body as an energy source (Backhed et al., 2005) as well having the ability to increase the number of T cells you have to fight infections.

Although you have your own unique microbiome, it is not fixed and can be changed. Probiotics which are live bacteria found in some foods naturally and also in supplements may benefit your health, as can increasing your fibre intake, depending on your normal diet. Fibre can have a direct effect on how the gut functions by adding bulk to the gut contents and reducing the risk of constipation, but it also has an indirect effect on health by influencing the gut microbiome.

Your microbiota and your gut immune system interact. The immune system is able to identify and destroy harmful bacteria while not destroying beneficial bacteria. Body composition may be influenced by the gut microbiota. Studies of those at higher weight have shown less variety in their microbiota. This is complicated because a low fibre, more energy-dense diet has also been linked to higher weight; however, there are specific species of bacteria which seem to rarely be present in those at higher weight (Valdes et al., 2018). Long-term weight gain has also been linked to less variety in people's microbiota (Menni et al., 2017).

Food choices can alter your microbiota, but there are other factors over which you have less control. Some medications, including antibiotics, can have an adverse effect on the gut microbiota, and it is worth considering taking a probiotic, or using foods to provide a source of more helpful bacteria after taking a course of antibiotics. Foods which naturally contain beneficial live bacteria include live yoghurt, kefir, sauerkraut and miso. There isn't enough evidence yet to say whether a supplement or food is the better source of Probiotics. Including both is very unlikely to cause harm, unless you have a significant medical condition where you are not advised to take probiotics at all.

Performance and the gut microbiome

Research in endurance athletes found that the gut microbiota may have a key role in controlling the oxidative stress and inflammatory responses to endurance exercise in the body, as well as improving metabolism and energy expenditure during intense exercise (Mach & Fuster-Botella, 2017). A low carbohydrate diet, which results in a lower fibre intake, has also been shown to result in more inflammation short term (Badenhorst et al., 2015).

The gut microbiome and brain function

There are link between brain function and the gut microbiota which will become clearer in the next few years. Research is showing fewer bacteria regarded as beneficial in those suffering mood disorders (Huang et al., 2019).

The links between gut microbes and health

Area of health	Impact of changes in gut microbes
Risk of getting gut disturbances	Providing your gut with a range of types of fibre can reduce the risk of gut upsets
Digestive problems during/after a course of antibiotics	Can kill off both beneficial and disease-causing bacteria. Probiotics can help minimise the problems often experienced
Mood and energy levels	Changing diet and/or taking probiotics to change the balance of bacteria in the bowel may impact on both mood and energy levels

III Irritable bowel syndrome

Irritable Bowel Syndrome (IBS) is a medical condition that has been estimated to affect around 4% of the population globally, with a higher proportion of sufferers being female rather than male (Oka et al., 2020). It is a condition that involves a collection of gut symptoms which include bloating, wind/gas, abdominal pain, constipation and/or diarrhoea. People with IBS have at least three of these symptoms, but always including abdominal pain, which can occur with unpredictable frequency. To be diagnosed with IBS symptoms need to be happening on average for at least one day each week for three months (Rome IV criteria), but of course even if the frequency is less, these symptoms can have a major impact on a dancer and their life.

The severity of symptoms varies from one person to another. If you start to suffer from gut symptoms including abdominal pain, a change in bowel habits and wind/gas, that you haven't experienced before and these last for six months, or less time than this if you are unable to undertake your normal dance schedule, please see your GP. As the symptoms of pain/bloating and a change in bowel habit can be caused by a number of medical conditions, it is essential that tests are done to exclude other medical conditions that would require different treatment. These conditions would include coeliac disease and could include inflammation or infection in the gut, or RED-S. Hypermobility can also impact gut function and is important to take into account in diagnosis and treatment. Once IBS has been diagnosed then the information below is aimed at minimising symptoms.

For many people, there are triggers for their IBS, and avoiding these triggers can reduce the frequency of symptoms significantly. While some of these are related to food and drink, others are more lifestyle related. Because the gut contains many nerve endings, stress can make IBS worse, even when food and drink haven't been changed at all. Sometimes it can be related to changes in the amount eaten or the timing rather than the food itself.

Some practical tips include eating regularly, allowing enough time to chew food properly and ideally to relax after eating a meal. Dancers who have very busy schedules may find their best tactic is to eat smaller amounts more frequently, rather than have a larger meal then have to dance within 30 minutes or so. Splitting lunch into two, with a gap of a couple of hours in between each half, is an option that maintains nutrient intake but reduces the amount of food being digested at one time. This may not work with some schedules, but it is essential to find a way to get the equivalent to lunch and at least one snack in the hours between breakfast and dinner. Adequate fluid is, of course, necessary. Rather than fizzy drinks or regular tea/coffee, some herbal teas may help. Peppermint is known to help IBS, and peppermint tea can be soothing. Camomile and fennel teas are other options that some people find soothing.

The situation regarding the role of specific foods in IBS is not simple. While many people find that high fat meals, large amounts of caffeine, alcohol, fizzy drinks, highly processed foods and large amounts of fruit or fruit juices can trigger their IBS, making adjustments to these may not bring adequate reduction in the severity and frequency of symptoms. Some people find that lactose causes problems, in which case finding appropriate lactose-free alternatives can bring improvements. Others find that gluten is not well tolerated, and that naturally gluten-free substitutes such as gluten-free oats, rice, potatoes, sweet potato, quinoa and buckwheat, together with manu-factured gluten-free products such as gluten-free bread and pasta, bring an improvement sin well-being.

Sorbitol and xylitol are substances that many need to limit. They are used as an alternative to sugar in some sugar-free/reduced sugar products such as sugar-free chewing gum and sugar-free sweets. Both sorbitol and xylitol can have a laxative effect on anyone and some people are more sensitive than others. They can also cause bloating, so are best avoided or used with caution if you have IBS.

For many people making changes to their diet and lifestyle can resolve many of the symptoms of IBS. Increasing or decreasing the amounts and adjusting the types of fibre can reduce symptoms. If this isn't sufficient there is a further step that can be taken. There is a more complex dietary manip-ulation for IBS called the low FODMAP diet: the name is derived from the types of carbohydrate that are initially excluded in this programme. This diet initially excludes a significant range of foods, needs careful planning before starting and is only intended to be followed for around six to eight weeks. After this time if there is no reduction in symptoms, then all foods can be included again, and other options for managing the IBS will be ex-plored. If the low FODMAP diet does help reduce IBS symptoms, which it does in 50–80% of people, with evidence for efficacy only if supervised by a dietitian, then there is a re-introduction programme to follow (Staudacher & Whelan, 2017). This requires a further few weeks on the low FODMAP diet while different types of FODMAP are trialled in differing amounts to find out what each person can tolerate. As most high FODMAP foods are great sources of many nutrients, and FODMAPs themselves can contribute to healthy gut function it is crucial to follow the programme fully with the aim of excluding as few foods as possible for the long term.

It is also essential, if removing any foods or drinks from the diet, to be sure that the diet remains adequate for health and the dance workload. For this reason, if you do think that a low FODMAP diet might help you, then you are best to do this with a suitable qualified dietitian, via referral from your GP/family doctor.

If following current IBS dietary guidelines doesn't bring adequate relief of symptoms, and you are sure you are taking in adequate nutrition con-sistently, then it's worth investigating options for medications. There are medications that can help IBS that GPs can prescribe, but there are also some over-the-counter medications that can be useful. If you have been di-agnosed with IBS it can be helpful to ask your local pharmacist for advice on what is available. These options are likely to include ways to help manage pain, bloating, constipation, or diarrhoea, depending on which is the main symptom.

Probiotics can improve IBS symptoms. These could be from food, as discussed in Section 1, or from a supplement. There are many probiotic supplements which vary hugely in both content and price. There are some which have been well researched and there are good quality research data that they are helpful in IBS management. These probiotics tend to be significantly more expensive than other brands. Brands of probiotic where there has been little or no research to demonstrate they actually help are likely to be significantly cheaper. They may still be helpful: manufacturers will aim to include bacteria in combinations and amounts that are likely to benefit gut health. But there is an element of trial and error with brands where is little research, to see if they do actually bring benefits. You would be best to trial them for at least six weeks to see if they are helpful. Beneficial effects do seem to wear off over a few weeks after stopping them.

IBS research is ongoing, and it is a condition that is still poorly understood. Future research is likely to offer more finely tuned treatments that will offer symptom relief to more of those diagnosed each year.

IV Food allergies and food intolerances

Food allergies

Food allergies are serious medical conditions that affect a small number of the population. There is a lack of accurate data, but around 10% of babies and around 4% of children under five have food allergies. Most food allergies start in childhood, and while many children do grow out of food allergies, some do not. By adulthood, the estimated prevalence of food allergies is 1–2%. While some food allergies may be first diagnosed in adulthood, most will have existed since childhood. Research has shown that many more people – typically three to four times the actual number – believe they have food allergies than in fact do have one or more allergies when they are properly tested (Loh & Tang, 2018). Numbers of those with proven allergies have increased over recent years.

The main severe food allergies seen in adults are to peanuts and tree nuts, fish and shellfish. Food allergies typically require very careful attention to diet to avoid even traces of the food(s) that cause reactions. Allergic reactions to food typically arise very quickly after the allergen – the substance that causes the body to react – has been eaten or drunk. Symptoms include swelling of the lips/tongue/throat and difficulties breathing and can result in unconsciousness if adrenaline (epinephrine) is not taken quickly. Some people require a second injection and anyone who is prescribed an adrenaline auto-injector for severe allergies should keep two auto-injectors with them. If adrenaline treatment is required, then hospital follow-up for the next few hours is necessary.

While most allergic reactions are fast, often within a minute or so, some can take up to 24 hours or even longer. Slow reactions to foods make diagnosis a challenge, and if you think you are experiencing delayed onset allergic reactions to food, it is best to seek advice from a specialist allergy team to identify as far as possible the food (or foods) which cause a problem to avoid an overly restrictive diet.

There are now a number of food allergens that must legally be listed on food packaging in many countries of the world. Travelling dancers with allergies are advised to check whether the list in any country they are visiting is different to the list they are familiar with.

In the UK and Europe, there are currently 14 allergens that must be listed on manufactured foods. These are:

Celery
Cereals containing gluten such as wheat, rye, barley and oats*
Crustaceans such as prawns, crab, lobster
Eggs
Fish
Lupin: used as seeds or flour in some foods, e.g. bread and pastries
Milk and milk products such as yoghurt, cheese
Molluscs such as mussels and oysters
Mustard
Peanuts
Sesame
Soybeans
Sulphur dioxide and sulphites (used as preservatives in some foods)
Tree nuts, such as almonds, hazelnuts, walnuts, Brazil nuts, cashews, pecans, pistachios and macadamia nuts

*Oats may be contaminated with gluten during processing so must be declared. Gluten-free oats must also be declared as it is possible to be allergic to a protein specific to oats called avenin.

In the USA and Australia, the list to declare is currently only 9 of the 14 above: milk, eggs, fish, peanut, sesame, shellfish, soy, tree nuts and wheat. Readers with allergies are advised to check for updates before they travel.

Pollen food syndrome (PFS), which is also known as oral allergy syndrome, is a reaction to fruits, vegetables and nuts. It affects about 2% of the adult population. The symptoms are typically mild and include itching and swelling of the lips, mouth, tongue, throat and inside the ears, which starts within a few minutes of eating the allergic food. Typically, people with PFS react to apples, peaches, kiwi, hazelnuts and almonds, but any fruit/vegetables or nuts can cause a reaction. Many people find that if a fruit/vegetable/nut causes a problem when raw, then cooking it (including in a microwave) denatures the allergen and stops the reaction. Canned fruit/vegetables are also usually tolerated as canning involves heating the fruit/vegetables.

Dancers with food allergies have two challenges related to food. First, to keep safe by avoiding any food that could contain an allergen they react to. Second, to also get all the nutrients they require for a performance diet from the foods that they can safely consume. Depending on the foods to be avoided, this may require careful research and possibly support from a registered dietitian. As a starting point, we advise dancers with food allergies to check they are meeting their needs for macronutrients. For micronutrients, it's always useful to think about options for rich sources of calcium, iron, zinc and selenium.

Food intolerances

People who have an unpleasant reaction to food that isn't an allergic reaction have a food intolerance. Food intolerances can cause unpleasant symptoms but it is important not to mix up allergies with intolerances, as an allergy is potentially life-threatening, while an intolerance may be very unpleasant but not life-threatening.

True food allergies can be tested for medically while food intolerances, currently cannot be tested for.

In the general population, food intolerances are reported very commonly, and although data are varied, in some countries, over 50% of adults report an intolerance (Rentzos et al., 2019). In dancers, there is a lack of data, but anecdotally many dancers do avoid one or more foods, which will be impacting on their nutritional intake at some level. Because there is as yet no accurate reliable test, the only way to identify a problem food is to cut it out of the diet and then re-trial it, without changing any other factor. This process should be repeated three times if at all possible, and ideally without the person being tested knowing when they receive the suspect ingredient. It is possible to test for lactose intolerance with a breath test, which can be helpful for those who are unsure if this is causing them a problem. As the human body is very complex, and the digestive system has many nerves which can react to stress and anxiety, it is difficult to isolate items that are responsible for symptoms of intolerances.

As discussed above, while reactions to food intolerances are unpleasant, they are not life threatening which allergies are. However, cutting out foods, particularly a food group – perhaps dairy or wheat-containing foods, can have a very detrimental impact on nutrition unless alternatives are properly researched and included.

If you have a food intolerance aim to exclude the minimum number of foods possible. Often with a food intolerance – for example, lactose intolerance, which is very prevalent in some ethnic groups – a little of the food which triggers the intolerance can be tolerated without causing any symptoms. Those with lactose intolerance can usually tolerate a small amount of milk in a cup of tea or coffee, whereas a glass of milk would cause symptoms. The availability of lactose-free milk is very helpful for maintaining nutrient intake without causing symptoms in those with lactose intolerance. Those who find specific types of vegetables or fruits may trigger symptoms of IBS may be able to have small amounts with no problem. This is in complete contrast to a food allergy, where even a minute amount can precipitate a life-threatening reaction.

Intolerance to vasoactive amines is an intolerance where it is worth establishing whether small amounts of foods can be included. Vasoactive amines include histamine, tyramine and phenyl ethylamine. People who have an intolerance to any of these can suffer from symptoms that can appear to be more of an allergic response, such as headaches, rashes, flushing, itching, swelling, runny or blocked nose, irregular heartbeat, diarrhoea, nausea, vomiting or abdominal pain, which can start about 30 minutes after eating the food containing the amine (Maintz & Novak, 2007). As the list of foods with these amines is extensive, we suggest any dancer suffering from this intolerance seeks support from a suitably experienced registered dietitian.

Salicylates, found in aspirin and also in vegetables fruits, tea, coffee, herbs and spices and products made from these can cause a reaction in some people, although there is debate about how significant the impact of salicylates in foods is. Reactions to salicylates can be very wide ranging and include wheezing, nasal problems, skin problems and digestive problems. If you think you have a problem with salicylates its best to seek advice from your GP in the first instance.

Coeliac disease

Coeliac disease is not a true allergy and is often regarded as an intolerance to gluten. But it is in fact an autoimmune response and gluten will result in damage to the lining of the small intestine, and sometimes there are symptoms in other parts of the body, such as a skin rash. The treatment currently is a strict gluten-free diet, substituting foods containing gluten with naturally gluten-free or specially manufactured gluten-free foods. For example, potatoes, sweet potato, maize, rice, quinoa and buckwheat are all naturally gluten free. Oats do not contain gluten but some with coeliac disease react to a protein in oats that is similar to that in wheat/rye/barley, so need to avoid oats, although not necessarily permanently. Because some oat products such as oat cereals and oatcakes are made in factories where wheat cereals are made, there is a risk of contamination in the production process, even if no gluten-containing ingredients are used in the product itself. Any dancer with coeliac disease is advised to see a dietitian as soon as possible after diagnosis and then once or twice a year to check on the nutritional adequacy of their gluten-free diet and to make sure they are up to date with any changes in the diet, such as any implications from widespread food labelling changes. Because bone health can be affected by coeliac disease, and those on a gluten-free diet can struggle to meet their nutritional needs in some locations, dancers with coeliac disease need to take particular care to avoid RED-S.

V PCOS – polycystic ovary syndrome

Polycystic ovary syndrome, usually abbreviated to PCOS, is a condition which is very common, affecting around 4–20% of women of reproductive age worldwide (Deswal et al., 2020). Sign and symptoms typically start in the teens or early twenties. It can affect dancers, but it is important to be aware that sometime PCOS is wrongly diagnosed in dancers experiencing low energy availability (LEA) (see Chapter 11), as periods can be erratic or stop in both cases. But blood tests and an ultrasound scan of the ovaries can usually separate the two. The only time there can be difficulty in distinguishing LEA from PCOS is when a dancer has improved their energy intake so is no longer in LEA, and hormone levels can fluctuate as the body restores normal functions. If this is the situation you find yourself in and you are receiving medical care for erratic periods, then it will be easiest for doctors to make the right diagnosis if you explain clearly your current situation.

The three main features of PCOS are:

1   Irregular periods
2   Excess androgen levels: the 'male' hormones in your body, which may cause physical signs such as excess facial or body hair. It is useful to note that all women need some level of androgens, just as all men have oestrogen in their body, it is the relative amounts that varies between the sexes.
3   Polycystic ovaries – the ovaries become enlarged and contain many fluid-filled sacs (follicles) that surround the eggs.

In addition many women with PCOS experience weight gain and oily skin or acne and may experience thinning hair and hair loss from the head.

There may be a link between those who experience PCOS and those who experience disordered eating and eating disorders, more data is needed, but if you are experiencing both it is helpful that those who are treating either condition are aware of the situation.

Insulin resistance, which results in very high levels of insulin in the body, is commonly seen in PCOS, which leads to increased hunger and weight gain. The high levels of insulin affect the ovaries, resulting in increased androgen testosterone levels and no ovulation.

Treatment of PCOS

Medical treatment may be offered to help manage irregular periods and excessive hair growth/hair loss. Insulin resistance can be helped by adjusting the diet, particularly looking at reducing the glycaemic index of carbohydrate foods and meals, and reviewing the glycaemic load of meals and snacks, see Chapter 4 for more information on this.

Some doctors will offer treatment for insulin resistance with a medication called Metformin which is used to treat Type 2 diabetes. Metformin has been shown to help control symptoms of PCOS, but there is no consensus among doctors over its use currently. A review by Luque-Ramirez et al. (2018) concluded that a combination of medications including Metformin offered the best outcome for normalising blood glucose levels and weight, although research is ongoing with other products such as myo-inositol.

VI Diabetes – with a focus on Type 1 diabetes

Introduction

Diabetes – or to use the correct medical term diabetes mellitus (DM) – is a lack of the hormone insulin in the body. This can be a total lack of insulin which is the case in Type 1 also known as insulin-dependent diabetes, or a relative or partial lack of insulin, which is the case in Type 2 diabetes, and gestational diabetes. Insulin is produced in the pancreas, and its role is to facilitate the transport of glucose from the bloodstream into the cells for use as fuel. In doing this it reduces the levels of glucose in the blood. Glucagon, another hormone produced by the pancreas, normally ensures that our blood glucose levels don't drop too low.

There are other, more rare, types of DM which are due to medication such as high-dose steroid medication, the result of damage to the pancreas from another illness, or due to rare genetic disorders. One of those caused by a genetic disorder is MODY: maturity-onset diabetes of the young. MODY can vary in severity and can look like either Type 1 or Type 2 DM and starts by the age of 25.

There is another completely different types of diabetes which is very rare: diabetes insipidus, which is a very different medical problem and has nothing to do with insulin or glucose.

For simplicity, we will use the word 'diabetes' in this book to mean DM.

Type 1 diabetes, where the pancreas ceases to produce any or almost any insulin, usually starts in childhood or adolescence, sometimes in young adults but rarely over the age of 40. It is a serious lifelong medical condition, but one where effective management minimises the risks to health. Currently, there is no cure, although scientists are constantly researching options. A pancreatic transplant might sound like an option, but unfortunately currently, it is risky and the side effects are significant. There is still no clear reason why Type 1 diabetes develops, but it is not due to diet or lifestyle.

Type 2 diabetes is where the body produces inadequate insulin, but also typically there is resistance to the working of the insulin in the body. Type 2 diabetes typically starts in middle age or older. Some ethnic groups have an increased risk of Type 2 diabetes, and being at high weight increases the risk. For some people at high weight, if they lose weight their diabetes goes into remission.

There is a third type of diabetes called gestational diabetes which is seen in pregnancy. Pregnancy usually results in a level of insulin resistance, where the insulin becomes less effective at transferring glucose from the blood stream into the cells.

For most pregnant women, the insulin resistance they experience causes no problems, and they will be unaware of it, but in a small percentage of pregnant women blood sugar levels rise to a level which is known to cause harm to the body, and gestational diabetes is diagnosed. Screening tests are done in pregnancy to identify anyone with gestational diabetes, because there are medical and health consequences for the baby and mother if the blood sugar levels are not controlled to keep them within a healthy range.

Gestational diabetes is normally diagnosed in middle or late pregnancy. Because blood sugar travels through the placenta to the baby, it's important to control gestational diabetes to support normal growth and development for the baby.

Gestational diabetes usually goes away after the baby is born. But up to 10% of women who have gestational diabetes develop Type 2 diabetes later in life.

If gestational diabetes isn't controlled the health risks are greater for the baby than the mother. A baby might have unusual weight gain before birth, trouble breathing at birth, or a higher risk of obesity and diabetes later in life. The mother might need a caesarean section because of an overly large baby, and they are at risk of the medical consequences of poorly controlled diabetes.

Management of Type 1 diabetes

Insulin is the medication which is essential in Type 1 diabetes. Insulin lowers blood glucose levels and is given either via regular injections or an insulin pump. In addition having a means to monitor blood glucose levels is a vital part of diabetes control and can give valuable information, particularly to dancers. The aim of diabetes management is to balance the intake of carbohydrates from food with enough insulin to keep blood glucose levels in a range where they are neither too high nor too low. High levels over time can result in damage to the body, while low levels cause energy levels and brain function to temporarily dip and impact the ability to dance. There are now flash glucose monitoring systems and continuous glucose monitors available that can give updates on blood glucose levels as needed, rather than having to do a separate finger prick blood test every time. For dancers with Type 1 diabetes there is no doubt that this ability to check blood glucose levels can be a real benefit to maintaining good control. The multiple updates possible over a day will allow greater understanding of the effects of different types/amounts/combinations of foods, particularly carbohydrate choices, on blood glucose levels. Management of Type 1 diabetes consists of eating adequate carbs spread out over meals and usually snacks, balanced with enough insulin to enable the body to use the carbohydrate. If insufficient insulin is used then blood glucose levels will run high with consequences of low energy levels and often increased urine production as the body tries to get rid of the excess glucose in the blood.

Those with Type 2 diabetes may manage their blood glucose levels by adjustments to diet with or without medication, which can include insulin if necessary, to supplement the amount their body is able to produce.

For those without diabetes, fasting blood glucose levels normally range from around 3.5 to 5.5 mmol/l (Guemes et al., 2016). Symptoms of hypoglycaemia, low blood glucose levels, usually start as blood glucose drops below about 3.0 mmol/l (Cryer et al., 2009). Those with diabetes may experience symptoms of hypoglycaemia at higher levels than 3 mmol/l if their blood sugar levels frequently run at higher than normal levels. After meals, blood glucose levels can go up to just under 8 mmol/l for those without diabetes. Day to day those with diabetes are advised to aim for blood glucose levels between about 4 and 7–9 mmol/l. For those working in mg/dl the conversion factor is to take the blood glucose in mmol/l and divide by 0.0555. Keeping blood glucose levels in a very narrow range, for example, 4–7 mmol/l, is possible, but often requires considerable focus on testing, and adjusting insulin doses. Managing blood glucose levels is made more complicated by the impact of factors other than food. Exercise will usually cause blood glucose levels to drop faster than at rest due to the increased need for fuel for the exercise. In contrast, in diabetes, illness and stress often cause higher than normal blood glucose levels. Drinking alcohol can have variable effects depending on the amount and type and also food eaten at the same time. Some medications can impact on blood glucose levels as can hormonal fluctuations, particularly during the female menstrual cycle.

Running high blood glucose levels (over 10 mmol/l) in diabetes is not great for energy and performance short term, or health long term. For sure it is a challenge to keep blood glucose levels under tight control, but the problem with diabetes is that trying to ignore it will usually result in very erratic blood glucose levels, which may be too low or too high. As glucose levels drop in hypoglycaemia if nothing is done to correct them, there is a risk of fainting, and in milder scenarios reduced concentration and energy. High blood glucose levels will result in low energy, increased thirst and urine production in the short term, and risk damage to circulation, nerves, eyes and kidneys over the longer term.

The good news is that a meal plan for the dancer with Type 1 diabetes is almost the same as the recommendations for the dancer without diabetes. Including three meals spread over the day, with carbs, protein, some fats and vegetables/salad/fruit, with snacks as needed between meals is no different for any dancer. The challenge for the dancer with Type 1 diabetes is that they are usually best able to regulate blood glucose levels by counting carbohydrates. This involves learning how much carb is in foods and, using a formula of their own personal carb: insulin ratio, then being able to estimate the insulin dose required to balance the food.

Dancers with Type 1 diabetes will be anxious to avoid episodes of hypoglycaemia, usually referred to as a 'hypo'. Normally, when blood glucose levels drop, glucagon is released by the pancreas, which results in a rise in blood glucose to prevent hypoglycaemia, but when insulin is used medicinally it is not as fine-tuned as the non-diabetic system, and further steps are needed to treat hypo episodes. This is usually to take around 15–20 g rapid action carb, such as a 200-ml fruit juice or another drink with sugar in, or five to seven dextrose tablets or five jelly babies, followed by around 15–20 g of a slower-acting carbohydrate. This could be some bread or a sandwich, some fruit, a bowl of cereal, some crackers or a bar. Some people find they experience severe hypos, requiring glucagon injections, or night hypos, which disturb sleep. If this happens then a review with their diabetes specialist team is advised. There are different types of insulin, with different peaks and durations of action and a specialist team are best able to advise on this.

VII Post-COVID/other viral illnesses

Viral illnesses have long been known to be demanding on the body, and also that there can be longer-term fatigue after a viral infection. Research has struggled to produce any treatments for those with long-term post-viral symptoms. One large family of viruses is the Coronaviruses which can cause illnesses ranging from the common cold to more severe diseases. In humans, in 2020, a global pandemic was caused by a new virus, a Coronavirus known as the Sars-CoV-2 virus, which swept across the world. Many dancers caught COVID-19 from the year 2020 onwards. Unfortunately, recovery for some was not straightforward, as the virus left many people with symptoms that didn't resolve after a few weeks but continued for many months or even longer. The diagnosis of long COVID-19 was given to those with persisting symptoms after they had recovered from the viral infection itself. Just as COVID-19 affected people's health in many different ways, so too has long COVID-19.

The symptoms which have been described in long COVID-19 include those relating to extreme lack of energy and loss of strength, coughing, chest tightness and shortness of breath, problems with memory and concentration, dizziness and palpitations, taste changes, gut symptoms including poor appetite and gut disturbances and disturbed sleep patterns. Skin rashes unrelated to food but linked to exercise can also be a problem.

There can be a two way interaction between post-viral symptoms and nutrition. Shortness of breath will potentially be worsened be eating, as it's not possible to eat and breathe at the same time. The result can be that food intake is reduced to prioritise oxygen delivery to the body. The symptoms of long COVID-19 can result in reduced energy to shop and cook food and also reduced appetite resulting in nutritional needs not being met. Taste changes, or loss of taste or smell can reduce the appeal of food which may make it harder to eat enough.

Reduced nutrient intake may then impact further energy levels and strength, mood and concentration. Improving nutrition can't resolve symptoms not caused by deficiency, but good nutrition can prevent symptoms being worsened by poor food intake. Good options under these circumstances are to focus on foods which are more energy dense and easier to eat – needing less chewing, for example, or nutritious drinks based on full-fat milk or a higher protein plant substitute.

Long COVID-19 can have an impact on mental well-being, with symptoms such as disturbed sleep, low mood or depression and anxiety. Any of these can make it difficult to focus on having a varied adequate nutrition intake. For some people with long COVID-19 there is a risk of under-eating which will impact further on energy levels. For others boredom can result in over-eating, or this can be caused by emotional eating.

Managing when energy is low

- List foods that are good options for each meal – a list for each breakfast, lunch and dinner and a list of snacks.
- Use ready meals in the short term if necessary.
- Putting the options into a seven-day plan will mean that once the plan is made it can be repeated for the next week or two, until perhaps a second-week plan can be made.

Suggestions when eating is erratic and driven by emotion

- Plan meals and activities to go between meals, if normal dance activities are not possible for a period of time.
- Think about what can be done boredom/stress is bringing a risk of over-eating: activities that are not demanding but done seated, e.g., drawing, writing, knitting/sewing, or contacting friends or family for a chat can all allow the emotions that may result in over-eating to settle.

Suggestions for managing changes in taste and/or smell

There are five types of taste detected: sweet, salt, sour, bitter and umami – which is savoury. You may find that not all have been affected equally.

- Make notes of the tastes/smells you can identify, and which of these make food more enjoyable.
- Often adding strong flavours such as spices or sharp and bitter tastes like citrus can help.

- Use a variety of textures in each meal to make it more interesting even if you can't smell or taste much.
- Food served cold or at room temperature may be more appealing than hot meals.
- Smell training can be helpful: the charity AbScent has more information on this.

Not surprisingly there have been a number of suggestions for dietary changes that might help reduce long COVID-19 symptoms. One that there is currently a lack of evidence for is a low histamine diet, unless you do actually have an intolerance to histamine. The diet is restrictive and made more complicated as food can vary in its histamine content. Advice from a suitable experienced dietitian is advised if you felt this was an area that you wanted to explore. There are a number of useful Food Fact sheets available at www.bda.uk.com.

Nutrition after a viral illness

Nutrition after viral illnesses: challenges to nutrition	*Nutrition goals and strategies*
1. Reduced appetite	Opt for smaller more frequent meals or snacks. Milky drinks and milk shakes are useful ways of increasing intake when energy and appetite are poor. Smoothies that have a protein content from milk/yoghurt/nut butter are also useful: opt for fruit rather than veg and limit to two fruits per smoothie if digestion is an issue.
2. Loss of smell or taste	Work with textures to give variety, using different coloured fruits and veg (in small portions) can help meals look more appealing. If some aspects of taste/ smell are present use these to include foods that have more tastes (only if pleasant though!).
3. Immune system needing to combat bacterial and viral illnesses	Your immune system requires protein to function, together with enough energy from carbs and fats to be able to have adequate energy for this role
4. Low energy making shopping and cooking difficult	Use online deliveries if possible. Ready meals are useful if cooking is too challenging and when energy improves then batch cooking and freezing portions are helpful

---

VIII Resources

Verity – The UK PCOS Charity – Verity PCOS UK (verity-pcos.org.uk).
Diabetes and Sport (runsweet.com) advice and support for athletes with Diabetes, useful for dancers too.
Long COVID and Diet | British Dietetic Association (BDA).

https://www.plymouth.ac.uk/research/dietetics-and-health/covid-knowledge-hub.

IX Learning outcomes

After reading this chapter the reader should be able to:

1 Discuss the role of gut bacteria in health and performance.
2 Explain the difference between food allergy and food intolerance.
3 State options to help those with a poor appetite after viral illness to maintain their nutrition intake.
4 Review options for sufferers of IBS to minimise their symptoms during a dance day.

References

Backhed, F. et al. (2005) Host-bacterial mutualism in the human intestine, *Science*, 307(5717), pp.1915–1920.
Badenhorst, C.E. et al. (2015) Acute dietary carbohydrate manipulation and the subsequent inflammatory and hepcidin responses to exercise, *European Journal of Applied Physiology*, 115(12), pp.2521–2530.
Cryer, P.E. et al. (2009) Evaluation and management of adult hypoglycemic disorders: An endocrine society clinical practice guideline, *The Journal of Clinical Endocrinology & Metabolism,* 94(3), pp.709–728.
Deswal, R. et al. (2020) The prevalence of polycystic ovary syndrome: A brief systematic review, *Journal of Human Reproductive Sciences*, 13(4), pp.261.
Güemes, M., Rahman, S.A. and Hussain, K. (2016) What is a normal blood glucose? *Archives of Disease in Childhood*, 101(6), pp.569–574.
Huang, T. et al. (2019) Current understanding of gut microbiota in mood disorders: An update of human studies, *Frontiers in Genetics*, 10, pp.98.
Loh, W. and Tang, M.L. (2018) The epidemiology of food allergy in the global context, *International Journal of Environmental Research and Public Health*, 15(9), pp.2043.
Luque-Ramirez, M. et al. (2018) Combined oral contraceptives and/or antiandrogens versus insulin sensitizers for polycystic ovary syndrome: A systematic review and meta-analysis, *Human Reproduction Update*, 24(2), pp.225–241.
Mach, N. and Fuster-Botella, D. (2017) Endurance exercise and gut microbiota: A review, *Journal of Sport and Health Science*, 6(2), pp.179–197.
Maintz, L. and Novak, N. (2007) Histamine and histamine intolerance, *The American Journal of Clinical Nutrition*, 85(5), pp.1185–1196.
Menni, C. et al. (2017) Gut microbiome diversity and high-fibre intake are related to lower long-term weight gain, *International Journal of Obesity*, 41(7), pp.1099–1105.
Morgan, X.C. and Huttenhower, C. (2012) Chapter 12: Human microbiome analysis, *PLoS Computational Biology*, 8(12), pp.e1002808.
Oka, P. et al. (2020) Global prevalence of irritable bowel syndrome according to Rome III or IV criteria: A systematic review and meta-analysis, *The Lancet Gastroenterology & Hepatology*, 5(10), pp.908–917.

Rentzos, G. et al. (2019) Prevalence of food hypersensitivity in relation to IgE sensitisation to common food allergens among the general adult population in west Sweden, *Clinical and Translational Allergy*, 9(1), pp.1–10.

Staudacher, H.M. and Whelan, K. (2017) The low FODMAP diet: Recent advances in understanding its mechanisms and efficacy in IBS, *Gut,* 66(8), pp.1517–1527.

Valdes, A.M. et al. (2018) Role of the gut microbiota in nutrition and health, *British Medical Journal*, 361, pp.36–44.

Appendix A

Glossary of micronutrients: minerals and vitamins

Micronutrients

Vitamins and minerals are known as micronutrients because they are only needed in very small amounts in the diet, typically under1 gram or 1 milligram (mg) per day. Nonetheless, they are essential not just for performance, but for basic health and well-being. While it is rare to see deficiencies of some micronutrients, like Vitamin E, because it is abundant in foods and not difficult to absorb, other nutrients, like iron, can be much more of a challenge.

Micronutrients are best obtained from food in the first instance. Only if food choices do not include rich sources of one or more micronutrients are supplements useful to consider. Other than Vitamin D, avoid single vitamin or mineral supplement unless prescribed: it is likely that more than one micronutrient will be affected if food intake is limited, and a multivitamin/mineral with 100% of the recommended daily intake (RDI) or recommended daily amount (RDA) is advised. In the UK, the equivalent is the Reference Nutrient Intake (RNI), and in Europe, the Population Reference Intake (PRI).

In Table A.1, the RDAs for some minerals do not differ for males or females; for others, there are differences due to differences in physiology. Levels shown do not include any increases for pregnancy or lactation; any dancer looking for these is advised to check out the recommendations for their individual country. Readers under the age of 18 are advised to check the recommendations for their age group for their country; they will be similar to the figures below, but may be slightly higher or lower, depending on the nutrient.

RDAs are estimated to be enough for about 98% of the population, so there are a small number of people who will need more, just as there will be some people who will need less than the RDA. There are currently no quick, inexpensive and reliable ways to check whether you are getting all the micronutrients you need, though some can be tested for individually if deficiency is suspected.

Those who would find more information useful are directed to a review by Beck et al. (2021) which covers the micronutrients of most relevance to dancers. Many general nutrition textbooks will have more detail on individual micronutrients, which space here precludes. The US National Institutes of Health Office of Dietary Supplements has a comprehensive set of fact sheets on micronutrients that cover a range of information about each micronutrient, not specifically just about supplements.

Vitamins

Vitamins are a range of substances necessary for good health. They affect a variety of body functions, and, like minerals, are required only in trace quantities – milligrams (mg) or micrograms (mcg, μg). Most vitamins were first identified during the early part of the 20th century, between 1906 and 1939. Initially, each was given a letter, and then once the chemical structure was identified, each was given a name. Some vitamins are in fact groups of closely related compounds with similar physiological properties rather than single compounds.

Some vitamins are soluble in fats and are absorbed from the gut dissolved in lipids. These FAT SOLUBLE vitamins can be stored in the liver and so do not need to be eaten daily. A very low-fat diet brings a risk of fat-soluble vitamin deficiency in the medium to long term.

Other vitamins are soluble in water and are absorbed into the blood after being dissolved in water. These water-soluble vitamins are excreted in urine – excess cannot be stored, so need to be consumed regularly, usually daily.

Table A.2 shows information on the fat soluble vitamins needed by dancers.

Water-soluble vitamins

Nine water-soluble vitamins are essential for human health. Because they can't be stored, they are needed daily. Although they can't be stored, it is still possible to suffer unpleasant effects from large doses, and guidance on upper limits is given where possible.

As always, if possible it's best to get the vitamins you need from food, to benefit from the combinations of nutrients, and when looking at plant sources, the additional plant compounds that can benefit health. Table A.3 shows information on the water-soluble vitamins needed by dancers.

Table A.1 Minerals needed by dancers

Mineral	Good food sources	Role in the body	Recommended daily amount for adults per day, amalgamation of UK, USA, Europe and Australian/NZ data	Notes
Sodium	Salt; smoked/salted foods; some savoury canned foods (check labels); cheese, soy sauce	Neuromuscular transmission (nerve conduction); fluid and acid/base balance; regulating blood pressure	Acceptable range: 575–3500 mg	Those using salt in cooking and high salt foods, e.g., cheese, smoked fish, may meet their requirements from food; those who use little salt may benefit from electrolyte drinks/tablets containing salt*
Potassium	Fruit, vegetables, nuts, coffee, cereals, meat, milk, chocolate	Neuromuscular transmission (nerve conduction), fluid and acid-base balance; regulating blood pressure	Minimum 2000 mg per day, aim for more, around 3100–3500 mg	The potassium in fruits and vegetables is beneficial for dancers: aim for three portions of fruit daily**
Calcium	Milk, fortified milk alternatives, cheese, yoghurt, nuts and seeds, grains, green veg, dried fruit	Bone/tooth structure nerve conduction, blood clotting	700–800 mg Upper limit 2500	If you don't use dairy products, check your alternative
Iron	Red meat, eggs, cereals, green veg, pulses	Haemoglobin/myoglobin formation, immune system	Females:15+mg Males: 9 mg Upper limit 45 mg (unless medically prescribed)	Plant sources of iron are harder to absorb than animal sources: Vit C from fruit/veg can help absorption. Avoid tea/coffee for an hour on either side of meals as they significantly reduce iron absorption

(Continued)

Mineral	Good food sources	Role in the body	Recommended daily amount for adults per day, amalgamation of UK, USA, Europe and Australian/NZ data	Notes
Magnesium	Nuts and seeds, spinach wholegrains, pulses, cocoa, soy milk, meat, yoghurt	Neuromuscular transmission, bone formation, enzyme reactions – energy metabolism	Females 280 mg Males 350 mg Limit intake from supplements to 350 mg in total	Low magnesium intakes have been reported in dancers, aim to include good sources daily
Phosphorous	Dairy, salmon, chicken, meat grains, green veg,	Bone/tooth formation, energy metabolism	550–800 mg Upper limit 4000 mg	Low protein intakes will result in lower phosphorous intakes
Zinc	Meat, wheatgerm, seafood, seeds, nuts, wholegrains. Green veg provides moderate amounts	Enzyme synthesis, regulate mood Immune system, wound healing	Females 7–12 mg Males 9.5–15 mg Upper limit 40 mg	Low intakes have been reported in dancers, aim for a higher intake of zinc rich foods if your diet is mostly or completely plant based due to phytates which reduce availability
Copper	Shellfish, organ meat, pulses, nuts cocoa	Enzyme synthesis	1.2–3 mg Upper limit 10 mg	High doses of Zinc supplements reduce copper absorption
Iodine	Seafood, dairy, eggs, and salt in some countries	Thyroid function	130–150 mcg Upper limit 1100 mcg	If you live in a country such as the UK where most salt is not fortified then low intake is a risk if dairy/fish are excluded

	Sources	Function	Amount	Notes
Fluoride	Seafood, water, tea	Tooth structure	Not regarded as essential USA advises Females 3 mg Males 4 mg Upper limit 10 mg/day	Low intakes are linked with dental caries, but high intakes can cause bone disease. Black tea provides more than food, typically 1 mg from 2–3 cups
Manganese	Nuts, dried fruit, cereals, tea	Enzyme synthesis	Females 1.8–5 mg Males 2.3–5.5 mg	Lack of data, but high doses from supplements not advised
Chromium	Meat, dairy, eggs, fruit, vegetables, nuts	Glucose/insulin metabolism	Adequate intake: Females 25 mcg Males 30 mcg	Amounts in food depend on growing conditions and location. Vitamin C helps absorption, antacids reduce absorption
Selenium	Brazil nuts Seafood, offal, meat, grains	Antioxidant, electron transfer, mood regulation, immune function, metabolism	Females 60 mcg Males 75 mcg Upper limit 400 mcg	2–4 brazil nuts supply about 30–50 mcg, depending on soil conditions
Molybdenum	Pulses, grains, offal, nuts	Enzyme function	45 mcg	Deficiency rarely seen

* If at all possible use products that are tested by a recognised programme, e.g., Informed Sport (We Test You Trust).
** Dancers with severe kidney problems may have been advised it is necessary to limit their potassium intake
Mg = milligrams, mcg = micrograms, also sometimes written μg.

Table A.2 Fat soluble vitamins

Fat soluble vitamin	Good food sources	Role in the body	Recommended daily amount for adults per day; amalgamation of UK, USA, Europe and Australian/NZ data	Notes
Vitamin A: retinol (from animal products) and carotenes (from plant foods) which are split to form retinol in the gut	Retinol: whole milk, butter, cheese, egg yolk, liver (once per week maximum), some fatty fish Carotene, carrots, sweet potato, spinach, curly kale, cantaloupe melon	Normal eye function, especially in dim light, for the immune system to work effectively, for growth and development, keeping skin and body lining tissues healthy	All figures as retinol equivalents Females 600–800 mcg Males 700–1000 mcg Upper limit 3000 mcg from retinol Avoid high doses in pregnancy from food or supplements	Yellow, orange and red fruits and veg are great sources of beta carotene. It has 1/6 activity of retinol, but those eating a good range of fruit and veg will get 50%+ of their Vit A from fruit/veg
Vitamin D: Vit D3 is the form from animal products cholecalciferol Vit D2 is the plant form: mushrooms and yeats, also synthetic form, ergocalciferol (Vit D1 is a mix of D2 and D3)	Oily fish, liver, kidney, fortified foods such as spread, cereals, sometimes milk (check for your country)	Regulate calcium and phosphate metabolism. Bone health, immune function, injury risk and recovery Reduce inflammation Mental well-being	10–15 mcg (400–600 international units– i.u) Upper limit 80 mcg (3200 iu) unless prescribed: follow guidelines as excess is toxic	Aim to get 15 minutes sunlight without high-factor sunscreen between 11 am and 3 pm in summer months. Take supplements when this isn't possible

Vitamin E: Several different compounds, tocopherols and tocotrienols Recommendations given for alpha-tocopherol	Plant oils. Nuts and seeds Wheatgerm	Antioxidant, immune function	UK: Safe intake: Females 3 mg Males 4 mg USA and Europe: Females: 11–15 mg Males: 13–15 mg Upper limit 300 mg	Deficiency unlikely unless fat intake is very low
Vitamin K	Green leafy vegetables including broccoli, lettuce, cabbage Vegetable oils, cereal grains	Normal blood clotting, bone health	1 mcg/kg body weight	Bacteria in the gut can also make Vitamin K, so deficiency is rare in adults unless they have gut surgery or repeated antibiotics and poor diet

Table A.3 Water-soluble vitamins needed by dancers

Water-soluble vitamin	Good food sources	Role in the body	Recommended daily amount for adults per day, amalgamation of UK, USA, Europe and Australian/NZ data	Notes
Vitamin B1: Thiamin	Wholegrains, meat (especially pork), fish, yeast extract (Marmite, Vegemite), fortified cereals, beans, seeds, nuts	Metabolism of carbohydrates, fats and alcohol; normal cell function; healthy nervous system	Females 0.8–1.1 mg Males 1–1.2 mg Overdose unlikely though very high intake may cause nausea	Easily destroyed by heat. Deficiency unlikely if meeting carb and protein goals from food rather than supplements
Vitamin B2: Riboflavin	Yeast extract, liver, kidney milk, cheese, eggs, fortified cereals, lean meat, chicken, salmon, green veg, almonds	Energy production from macronutrients; cell function, growth and development	Females 1.1–1.6 mg Males 1.3–1.6 mg	Excess is excreted in urine: high doses in supplements not good value
Vitamin B3: Niacin: includes nicotinic acid and nicotinamide	Yeast extract, Meat, fish, wholegrain cereals, pulses	Energy production from macronutrients. Normal cell function	Females 14 mg Males 16 mg Upper limit 35 mg	Can be created from the amino acid tryptophan
Vitamin B6: 6 compounds including pyridoxine, the best known form	Poultry, fish, pork, eggs, liver and kidney, soybeans, oats, peanuts, walnuts and brown rice	Protein and carbohydrate metabolism. Normal red blood cell production. Hormone regulation	1.3 mg Upper limit 50 mg	Vitamin B6 as a supplement has been used to try and reduce symptoms of pre-menstrual syndrome: more good evidence is needed to advise as most trials use doses above upper recommended limits

Vitamin	Food sources	Function	Amount / limits	Notes
B12: Cobalamins. Cyanocobalamin is used in supplements	Foods of animal origin including milk, cheese, yoghurt. Fortified plant foods	Formation of normal red blood cells and DNA. Nervous system functioning. Intrinsic factor in the stomach is needed for B12 absorption	At least 1.5-2.4 mcg per day. No upper limits set due to lack of data	Those eating mostly or completely plant based need to use supplemented foods or take a supplement
Folate (natural form) and folic acid (supplement form) (sometimes known as B9)	Liver (avoid in pregnancy), dark green leafy veg, cereals, bread, nuts and fruit	Production of red blood cells, for heart health and to prevent neural tube defects in the foetus	200-400 mcg. Upper limit 1000 mcg	Females considering pregnancy are advised to take a supplement of 400 mcg until week 12 of pregnancy
Biotin (sometimes known as B7)	Liver, peanuts, nuts and seeds, tempeh, fish, eggs	Needed for fatty acid, amino acid and glucose metabolism	Adequate intake 30-40 mcg. Avoid taking more than 900 mcg	Eating raw eggs regularly can cause biotin deficiency
Pantothenic acid (sometimes known as Vitamin B5)	Plant and animal protein foods, some vegetables	Synthesis of Co-enzyme A needed for energy release from food	Adequate intake: females 4-5 mg, males 5-6 mg	
Vitamin C Ascorbic acid	Citrus fruit, peppers (capsicums), blackcurrants, kale, cabbage, berries, tomatoes. Most other fruit and veg are at least moderate sources, including potatoes	Wound healing: synthesis of collagen; antioxidant; helps iron absorption. Deficiency causes scurvy	Females 40-75 mg. Males 40-90 mg. Upper limit of 1000 mg advisable	Doses above 1000 mg can cause gut issues such as diarrhoea. Smokers need an additional 40% Vit C daily. Easily destroyed by heat: avoid overcooking vegetables

Reference

Beck KL, von Hurst PR, O'Brien WJ, Badenhorst CE. *Micronutrients and athletic performance: A review. Food and Chemical Toxicology.* 2021 Dec 1;158:112618.

Appendix B
Recipes

Recipes are given for 1–2 portions which can be multiplied to make more if that is useful for planning ahead to keep in the fridge or freezer. Always check and follow food safety guidelines on food storage. Please adjust portions to meet your requirements if necessary.

In the recipes, the following abbreviations are used:

Tbsp = Tablespoon (15 ml approx)   tsp = teaspoon (5 ml approx)

Nutrition Information for recipes (approximate)

Recipe name	Carb (g) per portion	Protein (g) per portion
1. Overnight oats	55	20
2. Granola in a pan	44	10
3. Eggs Shakshuka	48	20
4. Quick pancakes	47	9
5. Spanish Potato omelette	36	19
6. Burrito	48	31
7. Lentil soup	51	14
8. Omega rich salad	42	25
9. Stir-fry tofu	67	25
10. Multi-veg pasta bolognese (just the sauce)	22	18
11. Chilli	52	41
12. Shepherd's pie	52	35
13. Salmon tray bake	59	29
14. One pan Mediterranean style cod (with no couscous)	11	28
15. Hypotonic drink	2	0
16. Isotonic drink	4	0
17. 'Milk shake'	12	10
18. 'Smoothie'	31	11
19. Banana Bread	30	6
20. Mug cake	59	5
21. Muffin	23	3
22. Energy balls	8	2
23. Chocolate and Raspberry pots	22	12
24. Quick ice cream	28	2

Overnight Oats

SERVE WITH BERRIES AND BANANA

1 SERVING
5 MINUTES PREP + OVERNIGHT REST

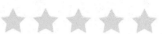

EASE OF PREP

INGREDIENTS

- 40 g oats
- 100 ml milk
- 2 tbsp Greek yoghurt
- 1 tsp cocoa powder or cinnamon (optional)
- 1 tsp linseeds or chia seeds

Toppings:
- 1 tsp peanut butter (optional)
- 2 tbsp berries
- 1 banana

DIRECTIONS

1. In a small bowl or container mix the oats with milk, yoghurt and cocoa powder. Leave in the fridge overnight or for at least 2 hours.
2. Once it's thick, add your toppings: peanut butter, berries and a sliced banana.

Add grated carrot, raisins and walnuts for a carrot cake flavor.

Credit: Pranch/Shutterstock.com

5-minute Granola in a Pan

SERVE WITH YOGHURT AND FRUITS

4 SERVING
5 MINUTES PREP + 15 MINUTES COOKING

EASE OF PREP

INGREDIENTS

- 160 g oats
- 80 g almonds
- 4 tbsp honey
- 2 tbsp vegetable oil
- 2 tbsp mixed seeds
- 1/2 glass water

To serve:
- Yogurt
- Fresh fruit

Optional:
- Chocolate chips
- Dried blueberries

DIRECTIONS

1. Roughly chop the almonds and mix with oats in a large bowl.
2. In the microwave or in a pan gently heat the honey until liquid.
3. Meanwhile, in a large pan add the almonds and oats.
4. Gently roast for 5 minutes.
5. To the pan add water, honey, seeds and oil and mix well.
6. Cook for further 10–15 minutes or until crunchy.
7. Once ready serve with fresh yogurt and fruit.

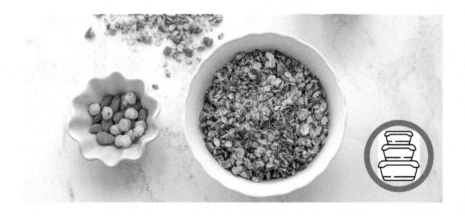

Traditional Shakshuka

WITH YOGHURT AND FLATBREADS

2 SERVINGS
5 MINUTES PREP + 25 MINUTES COOKING

EASE OF PREP

INGREDIENTS

- 1 × 400 g tin of tomatoes
- 2–3 eggs
- 2 sweet peppers (any colour)
- 1 onion
- 1 garlic clove/1 tbsp garlic puree
- 1 tsp olive oil
- 1 tsp ground cumin
- 1 tsp paprika
- ½ a bunch fresh/2 tsp dried parsley
- 1–2 flatbreads/pitta breads

Optional
- 2 tbsp natural/dairy-free yogurt

Vegan options
- Substitute eggs for crumbled tofu/chickpeas

DIRECTIONS

1. Peel and slice the onion and deseed and slice the peppers.
2. Put the onion into a small/medium non-stick frying pan with the garlic and a 1 tsp of oil, on a medium heat. Sprinkle over the cumin and paprika and cook for 3–5 minutes, or until the onions have softened slightly, stirring regularly.
3. Add the peppers to the pan and cook for 5–10 minutes, or until soft.
4. Tip in the tinned tomatoes, along with 1/4 a tin's worth of water (add more if it starts to dry out). Break the tomatoes up with a wooden spoon and stir in any seasoning (salt and pepper). Turn the heat down to low and leave to gently bubble for 8–10 minutes or until thickened and reduced.
5. Spread the veg mixture out evenly in the pan, then use the back of a spoon to create 2–3 little pockets. Crack an egg into each one, then cover with a lid or tin foil and cook for 3–5 minutes, or until the whites are set but the yolks are still runny (cook for longer, if you prefer).
6. Roughly chop the parsley, then scatter over, and dollop over the yogurt (if using) and serve with flatbreads/pitta breads.

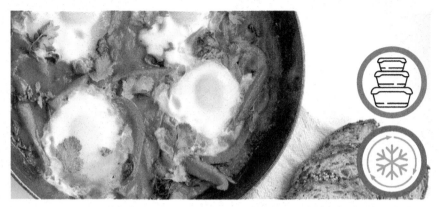

Credit: Arcady/Shutterstock.com

Quick Pancakes

SERVE WITH YOGHURT AND FRESH BERRIES

3 SERVINGS
5 MINUTES PREP + 10 COOKING

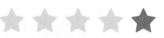

EASE OF PREP
Credit: KPPWC/Shutterstock.com

INGREDIENTS

- 2 ripe medium bananas
- 190 ml milk
- 150 g wholemeal flour
- 1 tsp baking powder
- 2 handfuls of blueberries
- Butter (or coconut oil for a vegan alternative) to grease the pan

Vegan options
- Substitute milk for soya drink

DIRECTIONS

1. In a bowl mash the bananas with a fork.
2. Add the milk and whisk well.
3. In another bowl sieve the flour with the baking powder and start adding this mix, little by little, to the mashed bananas and milk.
4. Combine well the ingredients.
5. Heat a knob of butter in a pan and pour the dough.
6. Add the blueberries on top of the pancakes and when they start bubbling flip them.
7. Keep going like this and add more butter/coconut oil to the pan if needed.

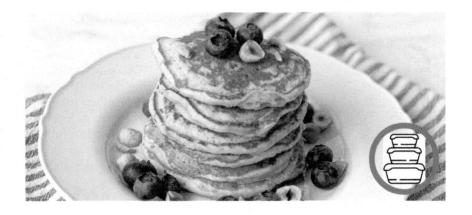

Spanish Potato Omelette

2 SERVINGS
5 MINUTES PREP + 40 MINUTES COOKING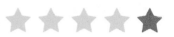

(20 MINUTES WITH PRE-COOKED POTATOES)

EASE OF PREP

INGREDIENTS

- 5 eggs
- 2 medium potatoes
- 1 small onion
- 2 tbsp oil, e.g olive or vegetable

Optional
- 1/2 pepper/capsicum, diced
- 1–2 tbsp cooked peas or other cooked vegetables of choice
- 2–3 tbsp chopped parsley or fresh coriander to serve
- Bread of choice
- Salad

DIRECTIONS

Before you start, make sure you have a saucepan lid that can just fit into your frying pan so you can use to flip the omelette.

1. Peel and cook potatoes: boil for around 20 minutes, allow to cool slightly then dice them. Peel and chop the onion.
2. Put the onion, and pepper if using, into a small/medium non-stick frying pan with 2 tbsp of oil, on a medium heat. Cook for 3–5 minutes, or until the onions have softened slightly, stirring regularly. Add the diced potato.
3. Beat the eggs and season with pepper and a little salt if liked. Add the eggs to the pan and tip the pan carefully to allow the egg mix to reach the bottom of the pan.
4. Every so often, move the eggs around the potatoes while it's cooking to ensure the eggs cook on the bottom. With your hand holding the lid, flip the tortilla onto the plate from the pan once most of the eggs has set. Then, slide the tortilla back into the pan carefully.
5. Keep cooking, gently shaking the pan occasionally, until completely cooked through.
6. To remove the tortilla from the pan, place a clean plate on top of the tortilla and flip again onto the plate. Garnish with parsley. Serve with salad and bread as liked.

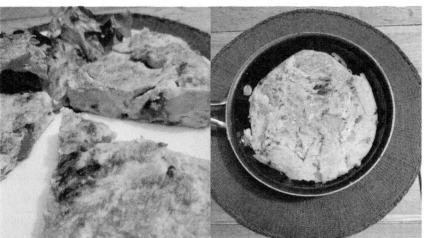

Chicken and Egg Burrito

WITH QUINOA AND AVOCADO

2 SERVINGS/2 WRAPS
5 MINUTES PREP + 7 MINUTES COOKING

EASE OF PREP

INGREDIENTS

- 2 tortilla wraps
- 90 g pre-cooked chicken
- 2 eggs
- 6 cherry tomatoes
- 1/2 pepper
- 1/2 avocado
- 1/2 pack of ready-to-eat quinoa
- 1 lime
- a pinch of salt
- a pinch of pepper

Vegan options
- Substitute eggs and chicken for crumbled tofu/chickpeas

DIRECTIONS

1. Bring a small pan to the boil and place in your two eggs for 7–8 minutes until hard boiled and then leave to cool on the side.
2. Cut the cherry tomatoes in half and roughly chop the avocado and pepper.
3. Once your eggs have cooled, de-shell and slice in half.
4. Lay the tortilla wraps out onto a big board/two plates and divide the quinoa between them, spreading it in the middle of the wrap.
5. Lay the sliced egg, peppers, cherry tomatoes, chicken and avocado over the top then add a good a squeeze of lime.
6. Fold the right and left sides of the wrap in to the middle and then roll up the wrap to the top to completely enclose the filling, press down the edge and then slice in half. Repeat with the other wrap. Serve immediately with extra lime and any condiments you like on the side.

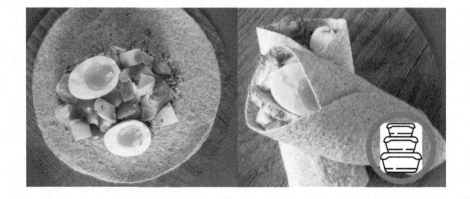

Lentil Soup

SERVE WITH BREAD OF CHOICE

4 SERVINGS
10 MINUTES PREP + 55 MINUTES COOKING

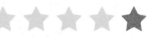

EASE OF PREP

INGREDIENTS

- 150 g red lentils
- 1 large or 2 medium potatoes
- 2–3 carrots
- 1 onion
- 2 tbsp oil e.g vegetable oil
- 1 litre vegetable stock (1–2 veg stock cubes)
- 1/4 tsp cayenne pepper

Optional
- 300 ml milk (to increase protein content and quality and give a creamier texture)

DIRECTIONS

1. Peel and slice the onion, and carrots; peel and dice the potato.
2. Heat the oil in a medium saucepan, on a medium heat for about 30 seconds then add the onion, cook, stirring, for 2–3 minutes, then add potato and carrot. Cook for a further 2–3 minutes stirring occasionally. Add the lentils, stir until well mixed in with the vegetables. Add the cayenne pepper and stir.
3. Add the stock and bring the soup back to the boil. Put a lid on the saucepan and turn the heat down until the soup just simmers.
4. Simmer for 45 minutes.
5. Add the milk if wanted, stir and reheat gently until about to simmer.
6. Turn off the heat. Serve, or for a smooth soup, allow the soup to cool until you can carefully blend it safely.
7. Serve with bread of choice (this adds protein to the meal as well as carbs)

NB To further improve the protein content of the meal, add a yoghurt to your meal.

Credit: Random Ilustrator/Shutterstock.com

Turn this recipe into a lentil dahl by adding turmeric and cumin and replacing half the stock with coconut milk.

Omega Rich Salad

2 SERVINGS   10 MINUTES PREP +
10 MINUTES COOKING

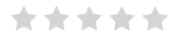

EASE OF PREP

INGREDIENTS

- 370 g quinoa, cooked
- 2 tomatoes, diced
- 1/4 red onion, diced
- 1/2 pepper (capsicum)
- 15 g mixed seeds (e.g. sunflower seeds)
- 15 g mixed nuts
- 2 eggs (omega 3 rich if possible)

Dressing
- 1 tbsp vegetable oil
- 1 tbsp soy sauce

Optional
- Apple/grapes/orange, diced
Vegan options
- Substitute the eggs with tofu

DIRECTIONS

1. Prepare the boiled eggs: place the eggs in the bottom of a saucepan. Fill the pan with cold water and bring the water to rapid boil over high heat. Once the water comes to a boil, lower the heat and cook the egg for 4–6 minutes.
2. In a large bowl, combine all the ingredients.
3. In a jar, add the vegetable oil and soy sauce. Cover with a lid and shake well to create a silky sauce.
4. Add the sauce to the salad and mix.
5. Serve with a portion of fruit to provide more carbohydrates.

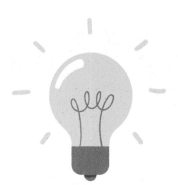

You can substitute quinoa with any other grain you have at home (e.g. rice, couscous, bulgur, etc.).

Stir Fry Tofu

WITH NOODLES AND VEGETABLES

2 SERVINGS   5 MINUTES PREP +
15 MINUTES COOKING

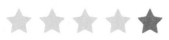

EASE OF PREP

INGREDIENTS

- 300 g tofu
- Egg noodles, 2 nests
- 2 medium/large courgettes
- 2 medium/large carrots, peeled
- 1 tbsp corn starch
- 2 tbsp light soy sauce
- 2 tbsp teriyaki sauce
- 2 tbsp olive oil or sesame oil
- Fresh grated ginger or ground ginger

Optional
- Fresh coriander
- Chilli flakes
- Sesame seeds

DIRECTIONS

1. Dice the tofu and add it into a bowl with corn starch, mix until the tofu is well coated.
2. Cut the vegetables using the "julienne" technique (or finely chop them if you don't have time).
3. Heat the olive oil in a non-stick pan and add the grated ginger. Stir fry for 1 minute (be careful not to burn it) then add the vegetables.
4. Stir fry for 5 minutes and add the soy sauce. Cook until soft but still firm.
5. Meanwhile cook the noodles accordingly to the pack instructions.
6. In another non-stick pan add the tofu (drizzle some olive oil if needed) cook the tofu and once there is a crispy crust add the teriyaki sauce with 1 tbsp of water. Stir well.
7. Serve your noodles with veggies, tofu and fresh coriander. Sprinkle some sesame seeds and chilli flakes for extra flavour.

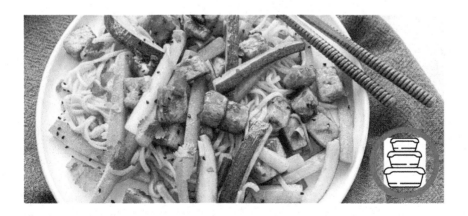

Multi Veg Pasta Bolognese

WITH PASTA AND GRATED CHEESE

4 SERVINGS   5 MINUTES PREP
+ 20 MINUTES COOKING

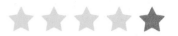

EASE OF PREP

INGREDIENTS

- 200 g pre-cooked lentils
- 200 g minced beef
- 500 ml tomato sauce
- 2 tbsp olive oil
- 2 big carrots, finely minced
- 2 celery sticks, finely minced
- 2 leeks, finely minced

Optional
- 2 bay leaves
- fresh basil
- parmesan

Vegan options
- Substitute minced beef with Quorn mince or extra lentils
- Substitute parmesan with vegan cheese

DIRECTIONS

1. Boil a pot of water and cook the pasta according to pack instructions.
2. In a mixer finely mince the carrot, celery and leeks.
3. Heat the olive oil in a large pan. Add the beef, vegetables and bay leaves and gently stir fry for a few minutes.
4. Add the lentils and combine the ingredients. Add the tomato sauce and season with salt and pepper. Cook for at least 15 minutes.
5. Serve with pasta, fresh basil and grated parmesan.

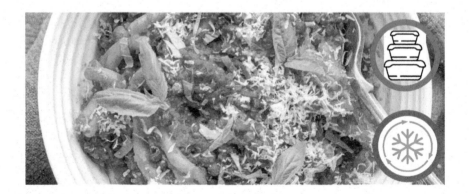

Chilli Con Carne

SERVED WITH RICE

2 SERVINGS   5 MINUTES PREP +
30 MINUTES COOKING

EASE OF PREP
Credit: Funstock/Shutterstock.com

INGREDIENTS

- 250 g pack lean minced beef
- 1 × 400 g can red kidney beans
- 1 × 227 g can chopped tomato
- 1/2 onion
- 1 garlic clove/1 tbsp garlic puree
- 1/2 red pepper
- 1 beef stock cube
- 1 tbsp olive oil
- 1/2 tbsp mild chilli powder
- 1 tsp ground cumin
- 1 tsp dried oregano

Serve with
- 60–75 g of rice per person or another source of carb

Vegan options
- Substitute minced beef for Quorn and beef stock for vegetable stock.

DIRECTIONS

1. Peel and chop the onion and garlic, and roughly chop the pepper. Drain and rinse the beans ready for later.
2. Heat the oil in a heavy-based pan over a medium-high heat, add the onions and garlic and fry for 5 minutes until soft. Add in the pepper and cook until softened.
3. Add the minced beef to the pan and fry for 5 minutes until browned. Add the spices and a little of the stock, fry for 1 minute then fry for a further minute. Add the chopped tomatoes and stock and stir to combine. Simmer gently uncovered for 30 minutes, stirring occasionally.
4. Meanwhile bring a pan of water to the boil, add the rice and cook for 25 minutes or according to the packet instructions.
5. Add the kidney beans to the chilli and cook for a further 5 minutes, until heated through. Season with salt and pepper and serve with the rice.

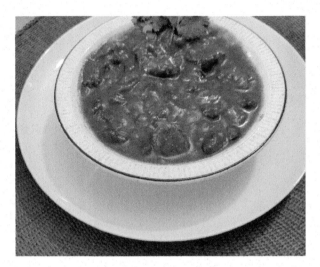

Chilli can also be made in a slow cooker or
pressure cooker with lean braising steak as
shown in the photo.

Shepherd's Pie

WITH VEGETABLES

4 SERVINGS   15 MINUTES PREP +
               1 HOUR COOKING

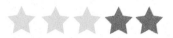

EASE OF PREP

INGREDIENTS

- 500 g minced beef
- 1 large onion, chopped
- 2 large carrots, chopped
- 500 ml beef stock
- 2 tbsp tomato purée (optional)
- 900 g white potatoes, chopped
- 1 tbsp olive oil
- 4 tbsp milk
- 70g spread

Vegan options
- Substitute the beef with 500 g Quorn minced or 250 g cooked lentils and 250 g Quorn minced
- Substitute milk with a dairy free alternative (i.e. soya milk)

DIRECTIONS

1. Heat the olive oil in a saucepan over medium heat. Add the chopped onion and carrots and soften for a few minutes.
2. Add the tomato purée (optional).
3. Once softened add the minced beef and crumble with a spoon and fry for 5 minutes, until the meat is lightly brown. Then add the stock and bring to a simmer, cover and cook for 40–45 minutes.
4. Meanwhile, heat the oven to 180°C/fan 160C°/gas 4.
5. Boil the potatoes for 10–15 minutes or until tender.
6. Drain and mash with 70 g spread and 4 tbsp milk.
7. Prepare an ovenproof dish, add the mince and top with the mush. Ruffle the mashed potatoes with a fork.
8. Bake for 20–25 minutes. (To bake from frozen, cook at 160°/fan 160°C/gas 3 for 1 hour or until piping hot in the centre.)
9. Serve the pie with roasted vegetables.

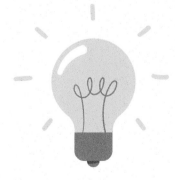

While cooking the pie, prepare a tray of mixed chopped vegetables (peppers, tomatoes, courgettes, aubergines, leeks, etc.) and bake for 30 minutes.

Roasted Salmon and Veg

2 SERVINGS   10 MINUTES PREP +
             30 MINUTES COOKING

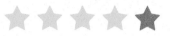

EASE OF PREP

INGREDIENTS

- 1 onion
- 1 pepper
- 1/2 courgette (zucchini)
- 1/2 aubergine (eggplant)
- 2 sweet potatoes
- 250 g cherry tomatoes on the vine
- 2 tbsp olive oil, plus extra to drizzle
- 2 salmon fillets (about 100–130 g each)
- Squeeze of lemon juice
- Handful of fresh basil leaves

Optional
- Swap the salmon for chicken, tofu, vegan sausages
- Add olives for a Mediterranean flavour

DIRECTIONS

1. Preheat the oven to 200°C/ fan180°C/gas 6.
2. Roughly chop the onion, pepper, courgette, aubergine and sweet potatoes into large chunks. Place into a large oven proof dish/ roasting tray and drizzle with the oil. Season as necessary.
3. Roast for 20 minutes, then add the vine tomatoes to the tray and lay the salmon fillets on top. Season with the lemon juice and return to the oven for 10–12 minutes until the salmon is just cooked through and the vegetables are tender. Scatter with fresh basil leaves to serve.

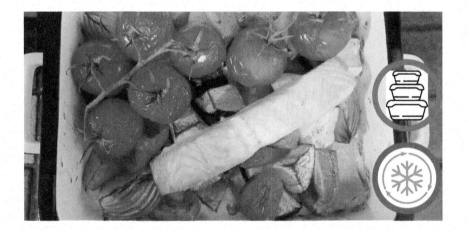

One Pan Mediterranean Style Cod

WITH COUSCOUS

2 SERVINGS   15 MINUTES PREP +
15 MINUTES COOKING

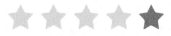

EASE OF PREP

INGREDIENTS

- 280 g cod (2 fillets)
- 250 g cherry tomatoes, halved
- 1 tbsp capers
- 30 g black olives, chopped
- 1 pepper (capsicum), chopped or 160 g frozen peppers
- 1 tbsp olive oil
- 1/2 small red onion, sliced
- 2 tbsp white flour
- 1 tsp dried oregano (optional)
- 1 tsp dried thyme (optional)

Vegan options
- Substitute the fish with plain tofu and follow the same instructions.

DIRECTIONS

1. Chop the cod into large chunks.
2. Add the cod and flour into a bowl and mix well.
3. In a pan, heat the olive oil over medium heat and add the capers, olives and dried herbs.
4. After a few minutes add the onion and cook for 5 minutes.
5. Add a dash of water if needed.
6. Once the onion is softer, add the chopped tomatoes and peppers and cook for further 10 minutes.
7. Once the cherry tomatoes are almost cooked, add the cod and cook for 10 minutes – be careful not to overcook.
8. Meanwhile, prepare the couscous following the packet instructions.
9. Serve with couscous as this will provide carbohydrates to your meal and additional protein.

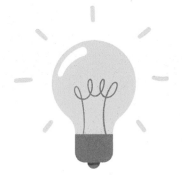

To turn this meal into a curry, add 1/2 glass of tomatoes sauce and a 1/2 glass of coconut meal. Serve with basmati rice.

Isotonic and Hypotonic Sports Drinks

2 SERVINGS   5 MINUTES PREP

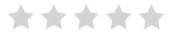

EASE OF PREP

INGREDIENTS

Isotonic

200 ml fruit squash		500 ml fruit juice
800 ml water	OR	500 ml water
1/4 tsp of salt		1/4 tsp of salt

Hypotonic

100 ml fruit squash		250 ml fruit juice
900 ml water	OR	750 ml water
1/4 tsp of salt		1/4 tsp of salt

DIRECTIONS

1. Mix all of the ingredients into a large jug and stir thoroughly.
2. Separate out into 2 × 500 ml or 1 × 1 l bottle(s). If not using that day then keep in the fridge until needed.

Isotonic drinks are great for a mix of rehydration and refuelling.

Hypotonic drinks are great for replenishing fluids quickly.

Post Exercise Chocolate Milk

1 SERVING   5 MINUTES PREP

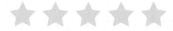

INGREDIENTS

- 250 ml milk/non-dairy milk
- 1 tbsp cocoa powder

Optional
- 1 tbsp almond butter
- 1 tbsp honey
- 1 small banana

DIRECTIONS

1. Combine the cocoa powder with a splash of milk in a glass and stir until smooth. Pour in the remaining milk.

Heat in the microwave or on the hob for a pre-sleep hot chocolate alternative.

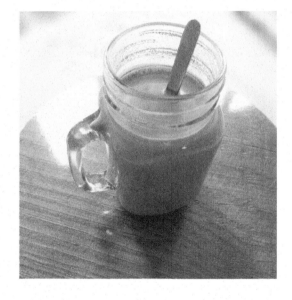

Banana and Blueberry Smoothie

1 SERVING   5 MINUTES PREP

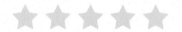

EASE OF PREP

INGREDIENTS

- 1 small banana
- 150 ml milk/non-dairy milk
- 1 tbsp porridge oats 10–12 blueberries
- 1 tsp honey/maple syrup
- 1 tsp vanilla extract
- 1 tbsp ground flaxseed, pinch ground cinnamon, handful spinach

Optional
- 1 tbsp almond butter
- 2 tbsp natural/dairy-free yogurt

DIRECTIONS

1. Put all the ingredients in a blender and whizz for 1 minute until smooth.
2. Pour the banana blueberry smoothie into one glass to serve.

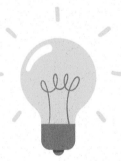

Can be stored in the fridge in a sealed container for 1 day.

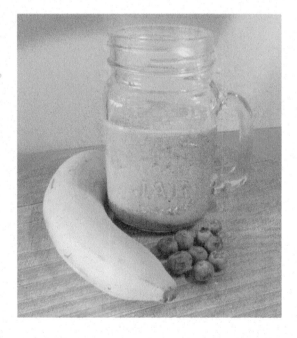

Banana Bread

SERVE WITH YOGHURT

12 SERVINGS   10 MINUTES PREP +
                  45 MINUTES COOKING

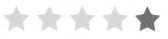

EASE OF PREP

INGREDIENTS

- 2 large ripe bananas
- 125 g wholegrain flour
- 125 g white flour
- 50 g buckwheat flour
- 3 tsp baking powder
- 80 g sugar
- 180 ml milk
- 50 ml sunflower oil
- 80 g of mixed nuts, seeds, chocolate or raisins

Optional
- Serve with 2 tbsp yogurt

Vegan options
- Substitute milk for soya drink

DIRECTIONS

1. Preheat the oven to 180°C.
2. Grease a loaf tin with some sunflower oil.
3. Mash bananas in a large bowl, add milk and sunflower oil.
4. To the same bowl add the three flours, baking powder and sugar. Combine the ingredients together.
5. Add the chopped nuts, chocolate chips or anything else you fancy.
6. Pour into the greased loaf tin and spread the dough evenly.
7. Sprinkle over extra toppings.
8. Bake for 45/50 minutes until a skewer inserted comes out clean.

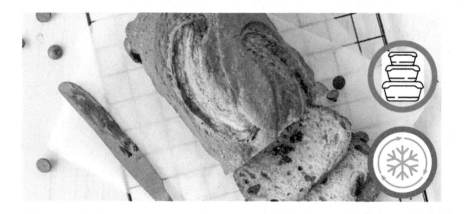

Blueberry Mug Cake

ADAPTABLE FOR DIFFERENT FLAVOURS

1 SERVING   5 MINUTES PREP +
              1 MINUTE COOKING

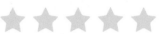

EASE OF PREP

INGREDIENTS

- 4 tbsp plain purpose flour
- 1/4 tsp baking powder
- 2 1/2 tsp sugar
- 3 tbsp milk
- 1/2 tbsp oil
- 1/4 tsp vanilla extract
- 10 blueberries

Optional extras/flavours
- Lemon zest/juice, ground ginger, cocoa powder, chocolate chips
- Serve with ice cream/frozen yoghurt

DIRECTIONS

1. Mix all the ingredients (except the blueberries) in a microwave-safe mug with a spoon until smooth. Then stir the blueberries into the batter.
2. Cook in the microwave for about 1 minute. If not quite cooked, continue in 15 seconds burst until cooked through. Let the cake cool for 1 minute before eating. Best served warm with some ice cream.

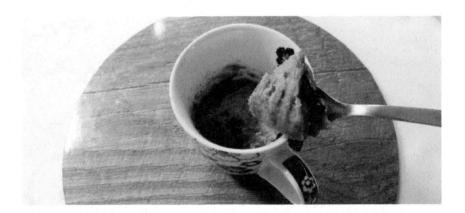

Breakfast/Snack Muffin

WITH YOGHURT AND BERRIES

6–12 SERVINGS   10 MINUTES PREP +
                 20 MINUTES COOKING

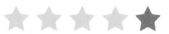

EASE OF PREP

INGREDIENTS

- 225 g yoghurt/non-dairy yoghurt
- 1 banana (small)
- 150 g golden caster sugar
- 150 g self-raising flour
- 2 tbsp ground flaxseed
- 6 tbsp water
- 15 g ground almond
- 1/2 tsp baking powder
- 2 tbsp maple syrup
- 1 tbsp mixed seeds
- 75 g raspberries

DIRECTIONS

1. Pre-heat the oven to 180°C/160°C fan and place 12 cake/muffin cases into muffin tray.
2. Mix the flaxseed with the water and leave for 5 minutes to create a flax "egg".
3. Beat the yoghurt with the oil and the flax "egg". Add in the dry ingredients (except the raspberries) and mix together until fully combined.
4. Finally fold through the raspberries and divide the mixture between the 12 cake cases.
5. Pop into the oven for 15–20 minutes or until a skewer comes out clean.

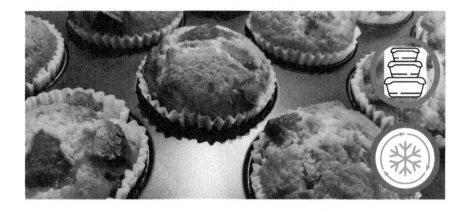

Energy Balls

ADAPTABLE FOR DIFFERENT FLAVOURS

2 SERVINGS   5 MINUTES PREP

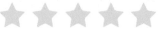

EASE OF PREP

INGREDIENTS

- 2 bananas
- 1 × 27 g sachet of instant oats
- 100 g desiccated coconut/ground almond
- 50 g nuts
- 50 g chia seeds/flaxseeds
- 50 g dark chocolate chips
- 2 tbsp maple syrup/honey

Optional flavours
- Ground cinnamon, ginger, vanilla extract etc.

DIRECTIONS

1. Crush the nuts into small chunks in a sandwich bag using the end of a rolling pin.
2. Peel and mash the bananas with a fork in a mixing bowl until smooth.
3. Add the oats, desiccated coconut, nuts, seeds, maple syrup/honey and chocolate chips to the banana.
4. Mix everything together with a spoon until it starts to come together.
5. Roll into approx. 16 small balls.

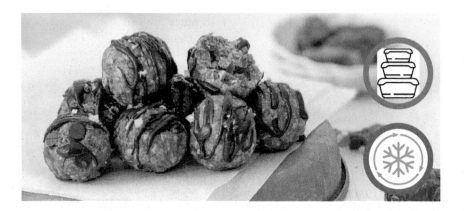

Chocolate Raspberry Dessert

2 SERVINGS   5 MINUTES PREP

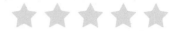

EASE OF PREP

INGREDIENTS

- 60 g chocolate
- 30 g raspberries
- 170 g Greek/non-dairy yoghurt
- 1 tbsp honey/maple syrup

Optional
- Chocolate sprinkles
- Any fruit can be used instead of raspberries

DIRECTIONS

1. Microwave the chocolate in a microwave safe bowl in 20 seconds burst until melted. Leave the chocolate to cool slightly.
2. Place the raspberries in two small ramekins or glasses.
3. Mix the chocolate with the yoghurt and honey and spoon the mixture over the raspberries and serve immediately.

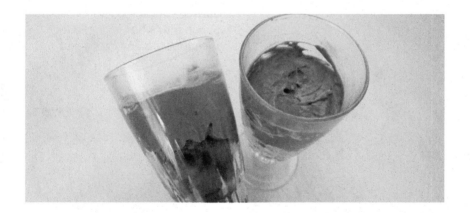

Easy Ice Cream

ADAPTABLE FOR DIFFERENT FLAVOURS

3 SERVINGS   5 MINUTES PREP +
              1 HOUR FREEZING TIME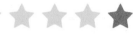

EASE OF PREP

INGREDIENTS

- 4 ripe bananas
- 3–4 tbsp milk

Optional
- Swap the milk for yoghurt
- To make sorbet, combine your frozen fruit with sugar and lemon juice

DIRECTIONS

1. Peel and slice the bananas and place on a cling film covered baking tray and cover with clingfilm.
2. Freeze for at least 1 hour, or until frozen through.
3. Whizz the banana in a food processor adding the milk between bursts until at the desired texture.
4. Scoop into 4 bowls or glasses, then top with any extras you fancy.

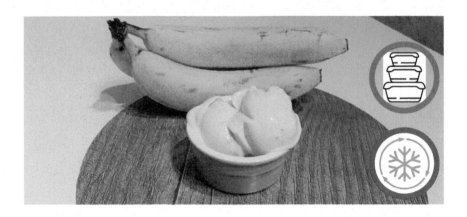

Glossary

All terms used in this book are explained in the relevant chapter: this glossary is brief and designed to be useful when moving between chapters where the same terms are used.

ATP   Adenosine triphosphate: the energy store of the cell

BCAA   Branch chain amino acids

Carb   Carbohydrate, macronutrient, source of energy, sugars, starches and fibre

Dehydration   The process of losing body water

Dietary supplement   A compound/food consumed additionally to normal intake to achieve a specific health and/or performance benefit

DPA   Docosahexaenoic acid: one of the omega-3 essential fatty acids

EFA   Essential fatty acids that humans need to consume from food

EIMD   Exercise induced muscle damage

Electrolytes   Substances that conduct electricity when dissolved in water and are essential for human health

EPA   Eicosapentaenoic acid: one of the omega-3 essential fatty acids

Ergogenic aid   A substance that may help performance

Euhydration   Fluid balance in the body

Fat/lipid   Mean the same, though fat is often used for dietary fat, a macronutrient, while lipid is used to mean fat needed by cells in the body for structure and function

Female athlete triad (The triad)   A combination of inadequate energy availability, low hormone levels and low bone density

Gut   The part of the digestive system that runs from the mouth, through the stomach and the intestines to the anus

Hypertonic   Fluids that contain a sugar content of 9+g per 100ml, higher levels of salts, or other particles for example proteins or fats.

Hypohydration   Reduced levels of body water

Hyponatraemia   Low levels of electrolytes, particularly sodium

Hypotonic   Fluids that contain fewer particles than body fluids and are absorbed relatively quickly.

Isotonic   Drinks that typically contain 4–8g carbohydrate per 100 ml, plus sodium, potassium and possibly other electrolytes such as calcium or magnesium. Macronutrients   the nutrients that can be used to produce energy

Microbiome   The combined genetic material of the microorganisms in the gut

Microbiota   The collection of microorganisms in the gut.

Micronutrients   Vitamins and minerals which are needed in small amounts for the body to function

Omega 3 fatty acids   Fatty acids needed in the diet as humans cannot synthesise them

Protein   a macronutrient required by the body for many structural purposes as well as functional roles such as in transport systems

RED-S   Relative Energy Deficiency in Sport – also applies to dance, and is where energy intake doesn't meet requirements

Trans fatty acids   Fatty acids with a chemical bond that is displaced from the natural form. Although they are unsaturated they behave more like saturated fats and bring health risks if not limited

Urea   a waste product of protein metabolism

Index

Note: **Bold** page numbers refer to tables and *italic* page numbers refer to figures.